Essential Yoga

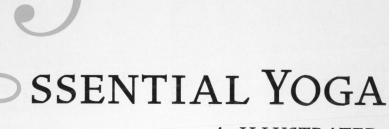

ESSENTIAL YOGA

An ILLUSTRATED GUIDE
to Over 100 Yoga Poses and Meditations

by OLIVIA H. MILLER

illustrations by NICOLE KAUFMAN

CHRONICLE BOOKS
SAN FRANCISCO

TO RUSTY, WHO LED THE WAY...

and in memory of Callie Tyber

Text copyright © 2003 Ohm Works
Illustrations copyright© 2003 Nicole Kaufman

Library of Congress Cataloging-in-Publication Data:

Miller, Olivia H.
   Essential yoga : an illustrated guide to over 100 yoga poses and
meditations / Olivia H. Miller.—1st ed.
      p. cm.
Includes bibliographical references and index.
   ISBN 0-8118-4115-4
   1. Yoga, Hatha. 2. Health. I. Title.
   RA781.7.M535 2003
   613.7'046—dc21
                        2003007881

Design by Chen Design
Illustrations by Nicole Kaufman
Manufactured in Singapore

Distributed in Canada by
Raincoast Books
9050 Shaughnessy Street
Vancouver, BC V6P 6E5

10 9 8 7 6 5 4 3 2 1

Chronicle Books LLC
85 Second Street
San Francisco, CA 94105

www.chroniclebooks.com

MANIFEST PLAINNESS,

EMBRACE SIMPLICITY,

REDUCE SELFISHNESS,

HAVE FEW DESIRES.

—*Lao-tzu*

Contents

CHAPTER 4: MEDITATIONS ‖ 135

CHAPTER 5: FLOWING ROUTINES ‖ 145

CHAPTER 6: YOGA SESSIONS ‖ 157

INTRODUCTION

GOD BLESS THE ROOTS! BODY AND SOUL ARE ONE.
—Theodore Roethke

Have you ever noticed that when you open a book about yoga, you often end up just *reading* about yoga instead of *doing* yoga? Many yoga books offer important and interesting information about the history of yoga, the philosophy of yoga, dietary regimes—basically everything you might have ever wanted to know about yoga. But when it comes to actually practicing yoga regularly, all that information tends to be less than useful.

This is where *Essential Yoga* comes in. It focuses on *doing* yoga. Designed specifically to get you up (or down!) on the mat, this reference guide is packed with over 100 poses and warm-ups as well as the basic information you need to do them. Detailed illustrations accompany concise, bulleted instructions, along with descriptions of the many physical, emotional, and spiritual benefits you will reap from a regular yoga practice. The simple instructions are accessible and easy to read, and you won't find lots of extraneous information. All this makes it easier for you to get down to business with a yoga routine.

Essential Yoga focuses solely on hatha yoga, known as "the yoga of activity." Hatha yoga is one of the most well-known and useful forms of yoga; it is the basis of many other styles of yoga such as Iyengar, Kripalu, Kundalini, Ashtanga, and Bikram, to name just a few. Hatha yoga originally developed as a way for ancient yogis (dedicated yoga practitioners) to prepare body and mind for the stillness, strength, and control required for a meditation practice. However, anyone can practice yoga, a system of personal growth and development achieved through postures, breathing, and concentration. A regular yoga practice promotes and helps maintain physical health, flexibility, and youthfulness as well as mental and emotional well-being.

Literally translated, the word *yoga* means "yoke" or "unite" and represents the union of mind and body. The Sanskrit word *hatha* means "union of the opposites": *ha* means "sun," while *tha* means "moon." It can also be translated as "determined effort," which is helpful not only when we're holding a pose but whenever determination and perseverance are required in other areas of our lives. Note that these and many other terms used in this book are in Sanskrit, an ancient Indian language that forms the basis of yogic literature.

A typical hatha yoga practice combines physical poses (*asanas*), breathing exercises (*pranayamas*), and meditations (*dhyanas*) as the pathways to balancing body, mind, and spirit. *Essential Yoga* takes these three key elements—postures, breathing, and meditation—and brings them together into a simple and complete reference guide for yoga practitioners and enthusiasts. The book is perfect for those who are new to yoga and want to learn more, for those who haven't done yoga in a while and need a refresher, and for seasoned practitioners who might want a review.

Essential Yoga is divided into 7 chapters: "Breathing Exercises," "Warm-Ups," "Yoga Poses," "Meditations," "Flowing Routines," "Yoga Sessions," and "Recommended Sequences." You may wish to start with a breathing exercise or two, choose a few warm-up exercises and as many yoga poses as you want, then wind down with a relaxing meditation and end by chanting the sound of *Om*. Or you can flip to the last chapter and follow any of the recommended sequences that fit your schedule, interest, and energy level.

Breathing Exercises

Chapter 1 features 12 breathing exercises, or *pranayamas*, designed to help decrease tension, increase energy, improve concentration, and promote physical and mental health. You may be familiar with the term *prana*, a Sanskrit word that translates as "life force energy," what is known in Chinese as *chi*. Prana "rides the wave of the breath"; it is distilled from the air that we breathe. *Pranayama*, then, is a means of controlling and extending the breath to regulate your physical and/or emotional state. Through yogic breathing, we can learn how to observe and become mindful of our breathing patterns.

Because breathing is so automatic, we rarely pay attention to it. Unfortunately, most of us have developed poor breathing habits over the years, only using a small percentage of our 5-quart lung capacity, leading to loss of energy, respiratory problems, mental confusion, and increased tension. If you really pay attention, chances are you'll find your inhalations and exhalations are shallow and that you tend to breathe high up in your chest.

Shallow breathing doesn't properly oxygenate the system, allowing toxins to build up. No wonder we often feel tired and sluggish by the end of the day. Full, deep breathing—also known as diaphragmatic breathing—floods the system with oxygen, nourishes the blood cells, and removes harmful toxins. The result is enhanced skin tone, better posture, fewer respiratory problems, higher levels of energy, improved concentration, and a feeling of overall well-being and health.

Our breath also controls our emotions. As we breathe, so we live. When we are angry or stressed, we breathe rapidly or may even hold our breath, which increases our tension level. Our muscles become tight and our pulse increases, which in turn shortens the breath, which increases tension, which shortens the breath . . . and on it goes. The next time you are tense, try to breathe deeply. With each slow, even breath, feel the tension begin to dissipate as your muscles relax. It is nearly impossible to remain in a state of heightened tension if your breath follows a long, rhythmic pattern.

The breathing exercises in chapter 1 will help promote this even, healthful breathing. Some exercises—like Complete Breath or Sufi Mother's Breath—can be done throughout the day: while you're waiting in line, working at your computer, or sitting in rush-hour traffic (breathe, breathe!). Don't wait to get onto the yoga mat to breathe correctly. Incorporate deep breathing into your daily routine and reap the benefits of increased metabolism, improved complexion, healthier lungs, a stronger immune system, better concentration, and reduced levels of stress.

Warm-Ups

Chapter 2 features 27 warm-ups, so important to any exercise regime. These warm-ups are designed to loosen your muscles and joints and to prepare your mind for the upcoming yoga session, helping you benefit more fully from your routine. Think of it as setting the mood.

Each page of this chapter features an illustration of the warm-up along with clear instructions and a list of benefits, including which parts of the body are targeted. Plan to do at least a few warm-ups before you start doing poses. Begin with your neck and shoulders, the places where we so often store tension. Move along the body and do a few warm-ups to awaken those hard-to-reach muscles along the sides of the torso. To engage the lower body, incorporate some leg stretches, especially to get those tight hamstrings and the muscles along the inner thighs loosened up. And, oh, that aching back! The twists, knee hugs, and stretches will align your spine and get your whole body ready for the upcoming poses. For ease of use, the warm-ups are alphabetized and categorized by type: standing, kneeling, sitting, supine (on your back), and prone (on your stomach).

Yoga Poses

Chapter 3, the longest chapter in the book, features 78 essential hatha yoga poses, or *asanas,* many of which have been used for centuries to promote relaxation, strength, flexibility, and overall health and well-being. *Asana* is a Sanskrit word that means "posture comfortably held." The chapter begins with tips on how to have a safe, effective yoga practice, followed by pages of beautifully illustrated poses with clear explanations, detailed instructions, and a summary of the physical, emotional, and spiritual benefits you will reap from doing these poses. As in the previous chapter, the poses are alphabetized and categorized by type. When appropriate, we've suggested counterposes that stretch, flex, and/or bend the body in

opposite directions. For example, Child pose (page 110), which curves the spine in a concave shape, is a great counterpose to the Bow (page 113), which bends the spine in the opposite direction.

Whenever possible we have included the Sanskrit name of the pose to emphasize the connection to yoga's ancient roots. Since *asana* is the Sanskrit word for pose, many of the poses end in *asana,* such as *Tadasana* (Mountain pose) or *Navasana* (Boat pose). The point is not to end up a Sanskrit scholar, but it may come in handy during a yoga class to know that the instructor means Hero pose when he or she says *Virasana.*

Whether you are doing yoga at home or in a class, it is not a competition either with others or with yourself. What is important is your willingness to focus within and attend to what is happening from one moment to the next. Yoga requires a very different energy from furtively checking to see who can hold the pose the longest, wishing you were more limber, or forcing yourself to stretch beyond your limit. The key is to do each pose slowly, paying attention to how you get in and out of it, how you hold it, how your body feels, and being aware of your breath. Aim for holding a pose in "effortless effort," where you feel the stretch, bend, or twist but are not straining or in pain. When you do yoga, your breath can be your greatest ally. The in-breath, *puraka,* is energizing; the out-breath, *rechaka,* is calming and balancing. With each inhalation, feel *prana,* or life force energy, infuse your body with vitality; with each exhalation, try to release a bit further into the pose. Direct the breath into an area of tightness and see if that prompts your mind to relax and your muscles to let go.

Remember that yoga is all about what feels right to *you.* Give yourself permission not to stretch as far as what is shown in the illustration. If necessary, hold a pose for a shorter amount of time than what is recommended. Conversely, you may wish to extend a pose if you feel strong enough. Tune into what works for you—your body and mind—at this moment in time.

Meditations

Chapter 4 focuses on meditation (*dhyana*), a process of quieting the mind and focusing on the present moment. This chapter recommends ways to introduce a regular meditation practice into your life. If you already meditate regularly, we hope the new meditations will add variety to your usual routine.

Choose from among 10 meditations designed to relax the body, calm the emotions, and still the mind. Meditation has been proven to reduce blood pressure, respiration, and heart rate; promote peace and serenity; and bring you into the present. Your entire being will feel calm, relaxed, and refreshed. There's only one catch: you have to do it. Many of us resist meditating because of the mistaken belief that we should be able to get on the mat, assume the position, close our eyes and . . . presto, start meditating. Unfortunately, what really happens is we get on the mat, assume the position, close our eyes . . . and start thinking about what's for dinner or that meeting tomorrow morning or those long-forgotten lyrics to some old '50s tune. It's easy to get discouraged and say, "I tried meditating, but I couldn't do it."

"Drunken monkey mind" is the wonderfully descriptive term for what happens when we try to meditate and our mind careens wildly from one thought to another, dragging our emotions and physical reactions along with it. Meditation is a way to slow and eventually still your monkey mind. But it takes practice and a willingness to suspend judgment and preconceived notions about meditation. Sitting in meditation does not mean flicking your thoughts off like a light switch. Our minds wander because that's what minds do.

Meditation allows us to take control and begin to rein in those thoughts. When you notice your mind wandering, instead of willing it (in vain) to stop, focus on your breath or a word or phrase from the meditation that you can use as a mantra—a repetitive statement to help you focus. As you inhale, try saying silently, "Breathing in"; as you exhale, say, "Breathing out." Repeat those simple statements as you focus on your breath; eventually the distractions that typically challenge your meditation practice will occur less frequently. And when they do occur, it will become easier to release them. Like clouds on a breezy day, let the thoughts drift by. Don't try to push them away or cling to them.

Flowing Routines

Chapter 5 features what is known as "linked" yoga poses, or *vinyasas*, done as a dynamic series with one pose following another. These 6 different routines allow you to move through your yoga practice in a rhythmic, flowing pattern. You can do a series slowly, or you may choose to pick up the pace, increasing your heart rate and providing yourself with a more intense workout. Some people find it helpful to incorporate a yoga series into their regular practice, because once the sequence is committed to memory, it is easier to establish a routine. We've included several different series from which to choose, depending on your time, stamina, and interest. Some of the routines also feature modifications for days when time and/or energy are in short supply.

Yoga Sessions and Recommended Sequences

Chapters 6 and 7 offer several complete yoga sessions and over 48 mini-sequences from which to choose. The 10 yoga sessions range from shorter sessions (20 to 30 minutes) to longer sessions (up to an hour and a half), depending on how much time and energy you have. Select one of the mini-sequences designed for practitioners of specific activities (such as dancing or bicycling) or one that focuses on a particular ailment or issue (such as back pain, allergies, or improving flexibility). All of them include thumbnail sketches of each posture along with references to the pages on which the pose instructions appear if further instruction is necessary.

General Recommendations

To assist with your practice of yoga—whether at home or in a class—we offer some general guidelines:

- Wait at least an hour after eating before you practice. If you're really hungry, it's okay to have a light snack (a half a cup of yogurt or an energy bar), but don't overdo it. You won't feel as comfortable or move as well with a full stomach.

- Drink enough water to ensure you are well hydrated, but as with eating, drinking too much will make you feel uncomfortable and have a negative effect on your yoga session.

- Wear loose, comfortable clothing made of fibers that breathe and allow you to bend and stretch with ease. You may want to dress in layers and remove outer garments (such as sweatshirts and socks) during the session and add back layers during relaxation when the body cools down.

- Many people like to use a mat when they do yoga. There are many types from which to choose—"sticky" mats that keep your feet from slipping and fuller mats that provide more of a cushion. You can also use a towel if you are practicing on a carpeted surface. In poses where your legs are widely separated, take off your socks and use a sticky mat so that your feet don't slip.

- Some yoga regimes require props such as bands, bolsters, blocks, and so on, but in general, you don't need a lot of special equipment, particularly if you're just getting started. Neckties, belts, and towels work as well as bands; a thick phonebook can take the place of a block; and a folded blanket can double as a bolster.

- As mentioned earlier, start your practice with a few warm-ups. It really helps to prepare your body and mind for the upcoming session.

- Some poses will instruct you to hold your hands in front of your chest at the heart center, palms together, in what is known as *Namasté*. *Namasté* is a Sanskrit greeting indicating reverence and honor and loosely translated means "I honor the divine in you" or "I greet the light in you." This salutation brings forth feelings of respect, acceptance, and openness.

- As a general rule, inhale when your body expands (lifts up) and exhale when your body contracts (moves down, bends, or twists). When moving into a backbend, for example, inhale; conversely, when going into a forward bend, exhale. If you get confused, breathe in whatever pattern feels comfortable for you. Don't hold your breath; the most important thing is to breathe. Don't get stuck on whether you're breathing "right" for a particular movement or pose. Unless directed otherwise, breathing is done through the nose.

- Follow the instructions and illustrations in the book but remember that the illustrations show the ideal, which may not be realistic for beginners, those with physical infirmities, or those who have not exercised in a long time. Some of us are naturally more flexible, while others are stronger. Do what feels right for you and your build. Remember that even simple poses can be deceptively effective and beneficial. Slow, steady progress is a safe and attainable goal.

- Relax into each pose. Don't strain or force, and definitely don't bounce! Stretch slowly and evenly. If you feel yourself "efforting" and your breath is rapid, you feel dizzy, or a pose simply hurts—stop. Come out of the pose and rest for a minute. Try the pose again if that feels right to you. Or skip it and try it again another time. Listen to your inner guidance.

- Don't stretch or bend to the point of pain or hold a pose to the point of weakness. If your muscles shake or if your breathing becomes rapid and uneven, back off of the pose or stop for a few moments and try it again (but only if you feel like it). If you feel any pain or dizziness, stop. Yoga should not cause discomfort.

- For poses that work alternate sides of the body, you will be instructed to work the right side first, which affects the ascending colon, then your left side, which affects the descending colon. This follows the workings of the digestive system.

- Make any adjustments you need to be comfortable. When lying on your back (supine), if you feel any back strain or your lower back arches, bend your knees or place a folded blanket under them. If your neck is uncomfortable, place a small pillow under your head so your chin is not poking above your forehead. When seated on the floor, lean against a wall if it is difficult to keep your back straight. You may wish to sit on a mat or firm cushion with your hips elevated above your knees, a more comfortable position for the lower back. Sit in a chair if it is easier and feels better. Make sure your spine is extended (lengthened); place your feet on a cushion to ensure that your knees and hips are level or that your knees are slightly higher than your hips.

- Balancing poses may be challenging at first. Try to focus on a spot on the floor a few feet in front of you. You will gain strength from keeping a soft, steady gaze. If you need assistance, hold onto the back of a chair or rest your palm against a wall. Your balance will improve with time. Breathe deeply and don't give up.

- Some poses include modifications to make the postures less or more challenging, depending on individual strength, flexibility, and energy. If a standing position is difficult, there is no need to skip a beneficial pose such as Mountain. Opt for Seated Mountain (page 92) and enjoy the same benefits.

- Advanced poses are also suggested for those who wish to perform a more strenuous version of a pose. Full Shoulderstand (page 131), for instance, is offered as an alternative to Half Shoulderstand (page 130); likewise, Proud Warrior (page 65) may be used as an advanced alternative to the Triangle (page 63).

- It is important to rest between poses. Some of the more energetic poses—such as Camel or Chair—flood your body with energy. Don't rush into the next pose; stop for a moment and enjoy the exhilarating energy coursing through your body. Other poses are designed to calm and relax—such as Child pose and Thunderbolt. Again, stop and from your center of peace and tranquility, feel tension ebb.

- Whether you are doing a breathing exercise, holding a pose, or meditating, concentrate on full, deep breaths. Doing so helps quiet the mind, balance the energies, and bring you into the present moment.

- Be sure to include time to relax in *Shavasana*, the Corpse, after you have completed the poses. This ancient pose allows your body and mind to fully absorb the benefits of your yoga session.

- Please note that not every exercise included in *Essential Yoga* is suitable or advisable for everyone. Before the instructions to each pose, we've noted contraindications (for example, people with hypertension or eye problems should not have the head lower than the heart). Please follow any cautions that may apply to you and always use common sense.

- Finally, be open to your practice, be gentle with yourself, and breathe deeply. Enjoy the many blessings that yoga welcomes into your life. *Namasté*.

Cautions/Disclaimer

Essential Yoga is not intended as a substitute for a certified yoga instructor or a yoga class. To find a class, talk to people who practice yoga about classes they have enjoyed. You can also check with health clubs, schools, or civic centers. Look in the newspaper for listings or check the Web. If you've never done yoga, it is a good idea to take an introductory class before simply diving in. Try different classes until you find an instructor and style of yoga with which you feel comfortable.

If you haven't exercised before, are pregnant or elderly, have a chronic condition, or have back or neck problems, please consult a medical practitioner before you begin. Don't do any pose that causes undue pain, shortness of breath, or dizziness. Not all exercises are suitable for everyone. Your physical condition and health are important factors in determining what's appropriate for you. This or any other exercise program may result in injury. The author, yoga consultant, illustrator, and publisher of this book disclaim any liability from any injury that may result from the use, proper or improper, of any exercise or advice contained in this book. Please consult your professional healthcare provider for information and advice on the suitability of your exercise program.

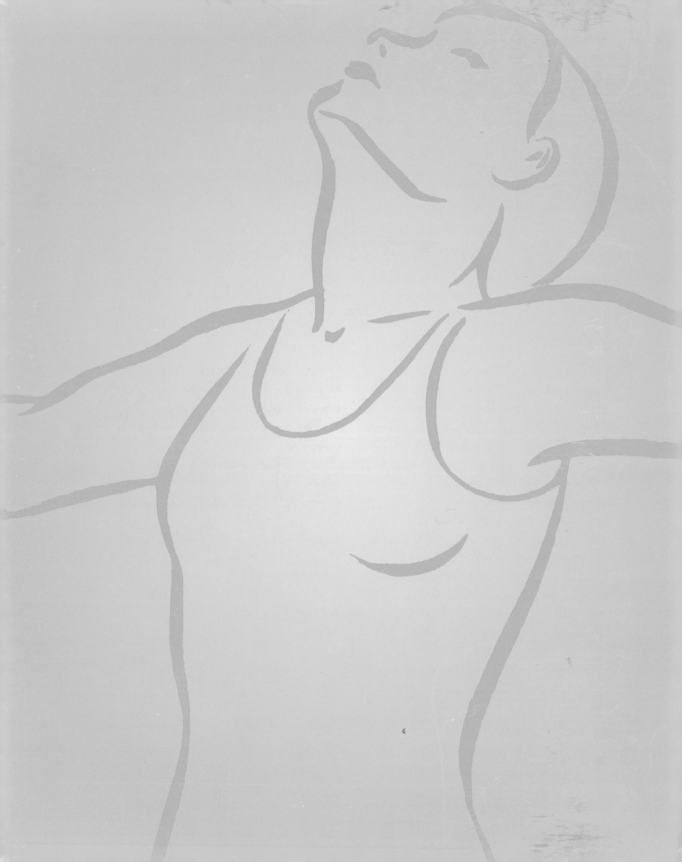

1

BREATHING EXERCISES

WHEREVER WE ARE WE HAVE THE CAPACITY TO ENJOY THE SUNSHINE,
THE PRESENCE OF EACH OTHER, THE WONDER OF OUR BREATHING.
—*Thich Nhat Hanh*

This chapter focuses on breath expansion and control, known as *pranayama*. The way we breathe has a profound effect on the quality of our lives. Our breath affects the body, mind, and emotions. Shallow breathing deprives the body of oxygen and the life-giving force, *prana*. When we breathe deeply, our respiratory, circulatory, digestive, and nervous systems function better. Our minds become clearer, and our concentration improves. Stress, anger, and tension dissipate.

Through a variety of breathing techniques, hatha yoga uses *pranayama* to help us more fully oxygenate and purify our bodies, to slow and calm our minds, to steady our emotions, and to balance our energies. The breath can be divided into four parts: inhalation (*puraka*), retention or holding the breath in (*kumbhaka*), exhalation (*rechaka*), and finally, suspension or holding the breath out (*bahya kumbhaka*). Inhalation brings nourishment and energy, holding the breath allows *prana* to fully enter and energize the body, exhalation cleanses the system and quiets the emotions, and suspension extends the benefits of exhalation

by further calming your entire being. Full, deep breathing that includes all four stages—inhalation, retention, exhalation, and suspension—properly fuels, energizes, cleanses, balances, and relaxes the entire system.

The 12 exercises included in this chapter encourage conscious yogic breathing, which engages the diaphragm, the large dome-shaped muscle that enables us to breathe. When we inhale, the diaphragm lowers into the abdominal area, drawing air into the lungs; when we exhale, the diaphragm rises up, pushing the air out. Diaphragmatic breathing allows us to fill our lungs completely, bringing in a fresh supply of oxygen, and then expel all the stale air as we exhale, promoting health and well-being.

Many of these breathing exercises include counting to help you slow and lengthen the breath and to encourage you to focus on your breathing. If you are new to *pranayama*, try to make your exhalation as long as your inhalation; eventually, see if you can slow your exhalation so that it lasts longer than the inhalation, an effective way to thoroughly calm your body and mind. The exhalation should also be longer than or equal to the retention of the breath that follows inhalation.

Most of these breathing exercises may be done from a supine position (lying on your back), in a comfortable seated position on a mat or a cushion on the floor, or seated in a chair. When in a seated position, allow your sitting bones to sink into the chair or cushion. Your pelvis is level, and your shoulders are relaxed and down away from the ears. Your chin is parallel to the floor and retracted slightly. Gently press out through the crown of your head. If you are seated in a chair, your knees may be slightly higher than or even with the hips; if they are not, place your feet on a cushion (see introduction to seated poses, page 89). If you are seated on the floor, you may wish to sit in Easy pose (page 90) or Half Lotus (page 90). Your eyes may be closed or downcast.

If any part of the exercise bothers you—if you'd rather not count, or if the count is too long or too short, for instance—make whatever adjustments you need. Some breathing exercises use sounds as a way to calm the body and mind. Although you may feel self-conscious, this is a great way to focus and concentrate on your breath. If you have trouble breathing or have a cold or bronchitis, wait until you feel better before you do any deep breathing exercises. If you suffer from heart disease or asthma, consult a physician first.

Before you begin, start by focusing on your "normal" breathing pattern. Sit or lie in a comfortable position. Close your eyes. Observe your breath. Try not to change or judge; simply observe. Does the pace of your breath seem rapid or slow? Is it even or uneven? Does your inhalation last longer than your exhalation? Do you hold your breath? What parts of your body move when you breathe? Do you notice any areas of tightness or tension? Do you breathe more from your chest or your belly? Do you breathe through your nose or mouth? Does observing your breath make you uncomfortable? Answers to some of these questions may not come right away; sit with them for a while and see what arises. Focusing on your breathing can also become a form of meditation, another way to focus and alleviate stress.

Once you become more familiar with your breathing pattern, the following exercises will help you explore ways to use your breath to feel stimulated or relaxed. As you breathe deeply, acknowledge the miracle of your breath—this amazing life-giving force that we so often take for granted.

ALTERNATE NOSTRIL BREATH

(*Anuloma Viloma*)

Although we may not be aware of it, we normally breathe in one- to two-hour cycles; first one nostril, then the other is dominant. (If you're curious, check which nostril is dominant by closing off one nostril and breathing through the other; reverse, and compare the airflow from each.) Prolonged breathing through one side can drain our energy. *Anuloma Viloma,* an ancient breathing technique, has a profound stilling effect on the mind and restores the proper balance to our breathing pattern, which equalizes the energies and pathways of the nervous system. Placing your index and middle fingers on your forehead stimulates the "third eye," our center of intuition and connection to the higher self. Practice Alternate Nostril Breath whenever you seek a calm, clear state of mind.

- Before you begin, you may wish to use a tissue to clear your nostrils. Sit comfortably in a chair or on a mat, keeping your spine straight.

- Place the index and middle fingers of your right hand on your forehead, between the eyebrows. Your thumb rests on the right nostril; the ring and baby fingers rest on your left nostril. If you prefer not to place your fingers on the forehead, curl the index and middle fingers toward the palm instead.

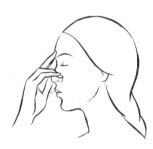

- Inhale and exhale. Close the right nostril with the thumb; inhale through the left nostril for a count of 5.

- Close both nostrils; hold your breath for a count of 5. (If holding the breath causes discomfort, reduce the count or eliminate altogether.)

- Lift the thumb; exhale for a count of 5 through the right nostril.

- Inhale through the right nostril for a count of 5, hold for a count of 5, close your right nostril, and exhale through the left nostril for a count of 5. This completes 1 round.

- Repeat for 4 more rounds.

EXPANSIVE BREATH

(*Phullana Pranayama*)

This rejuvenating, expansive breath opens the chest, promoting a sense of wellness and fulfillment. The movement also helps relieve tension in your back and keeps your spine flexible. Do this energetic breathing exercise when you feel cold, tired, or run down. It can also double as a warm-up to any yoga session.

- Stand with your feet about shoulder-width apart. Hold your arms straight out in front of you with palms together at chest height. Make sure your shoulders are down and away from the ears.

FIG. 1:

- Open your mouth and inhale through the mouth as you fling your arms open and back, bending the wrists so your fingertips point away from you. Lift the chin slightly. Your eyes look upward.

FIG. 2:

- Exhale completely through the mouth as you begin to come forward, tucking your chin, and bending at the waist and knees. Hands may be clasped together in front of the chest, or they may rest on your thighs.

- Let your head hang so that there is no pressure on your neck.

- Repeat this cycle 12 times at whatever pace feels best for you.

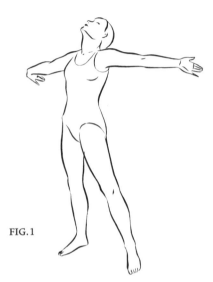

FIG. 1

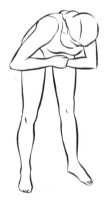

FIG. 2

BELLY AND CHEST BREATHING

(*Kuksa Pranayama / Uro Pranayama*)

Although this breathing exercise may be done from a seated position, it might be easier to feel the movement of your breath while lying on your back. Make sure you are comfortable so that you can attend to your breathing and not be distracted by discomfort in your neck or lower back. This exercise allows you to fully experience diaphragmatic breathing and purify and oxygenate your system. An added benefit is tension release and anxiety relief, resulting in a feeling of calm and serenity.

- Lie on your back (although you may sit if that is preferable). Place a blanket or bolster under your knees if you feel any strain in the lower back and a small pillow under your neck if you feel any tension at the back of your neck.

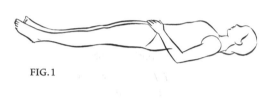

FIG. 1

FIG. 1:

- Close your eyes. Place your hands lightly on your belly. Focus your awareness there.

- Breathe in slowly. Feel your belly begin to expand and round. Your chest should not move. If you'd like, count to 5 as you inhale.

- Exhale slowly and feel your belly begin to flatten. If you'd like, count to 5 as you exhale.

- Rest for a few seconds and repeat 6 more times.

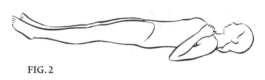

FIG. 2

FIG. 2:

- Move your hands so that they rest on your upper chest.

- Shift your attention to the middle of your chest. Inhale and imagine the breath expanding into the front, sides, and back of the chest. Feel your rib cage expand.

- Exhale completely.

- Continue breathing in this manner 6 more times, counting inhalations and exhalations if you wish.

- When you're done, compare how you felt when you did Belly Breathing with how you felt when you did Chest Breathing.

BREATH OF FIRE

(Kapalabhati)

Kapalabhati, an energizing and purifying breath, literally means "skull brightening." It aerates the entire system by greatly increasing the flow of oxygen throughout the body, tones the abdominal muscles, strengthens the diaphragm, increases energy, and helps improve concentration. Do not perform Breath of Fire or the raised thumbs alternative if you have high blood pressure, diabetes, or epilepsy or if you suffer from depression or insomnia. If you experience dizziness, consult a yoga teacher for guidance.

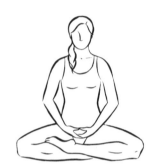

- Sit with your spine comfortably extended. Keep your eyes closed or downcast.

- Inhale.

- Exhale vigorously by pulling back your abdominal muscles. This will cause a short, forceful expulsion of air through the nose. Imagine that your exhalations could blow out the flame of a candle.

- Repeat with a steady, quick series of 20 exhalations.

- Stop and allow the breath to return to normal. Repeat with another set of 20 exhalations. Gradually increase to 3 sets of 20 exhalations.

BREATH OF FIRE WITH RAISED THUMBS

(Uditanguli Kapalabhati)

In addition to giving you all the benefits of Breath of Fire, *Kapalabhati* with arms and thumbs raised is a position of power that strengthens the energy center located at the solar plexus, between the navel and breastbone.

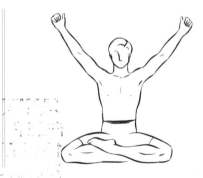

- Sit with your spine comfortably extended.

- Raise both arms above your head in a V position without bending them at the elbows. Palms face forward, fingers are lightly curled, and thumbs point in.

- Follow the directions for Breath of Fire.

- Lower your arms; breathe normally between sets.

CHIN PRESS BREATH

(*Murcha Pranayama*)

Chin Press Breath stimulates the thyroid, which regulates metabolism, while stretching the muscles at the back of the neck. It improves willpower and concentration and promotes a sense of inner peace. While doing *Murcha Pranayama*, focus on a goal you would like to meet, knowing that your steady breathing is moving you that much closer to accomplishing it.

- Sit with your spine comfortably extended. Close your eyes.

- Inhale through your nose for a count of 5. Lift your chest, moving your head back slightly as you tuck your chin toward your chest.

- Hold your breath for a count of 5. (Breath count may be modified to suit your comfort level.)

- Exhale through your nose for a count of 5.

- Raise your chin so that it's level with the floor.

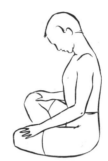

COMPLETE BREATH

(*Paripurna Pranayama*)

It has been said that the breath is the pulse of the mind. When we are tense, our breathing becomes rapid and shallow; this, in turn, heightens our tension level. Practicing Complete Breath will calm your emotions, relieve tension, relax your muscles, and help you concentrate. Complete Breath also purifies the respiratory system as you expel stale air from your lungs and oxygenate your blood cells. As an added benefit, deep breathing helps your complexion by increasing circulation and bringing more blood to the face. It's simple… just breathe (deeply). Relish the feeling of health and serenity that Complete Breath brings.

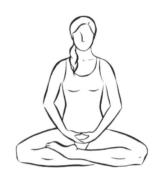

- This breathing exercise can be done in any comfortable seated position with the back straight, or in Corpse pose (page 127) with bolsters under your knees to keep the lower back on the floor and to prevent strain.

- Relax; close your eyes. If you like, you may rest one hand lightly on your chest and the other on your stomach.

- Exhale completely. Inhale slowly and begin sipping air in through your nose. Allow your stomach to expand like a balloon.

- Continue to sip in the breath, allowing the air to move into your chest, completely filling the lungs. Sip in one more breath.

- Hold your breath (retention) for a few moments. Begin exhaling slowly through the nose, down into the chest and abdomen, squeezing out all the stale air from the bottom of the lungs. Hold the breath out (suspension) for a moment.

- Repeat 5 times.

You may also wish to try a 4-part breath done in a series:
- Inhale for a count of 5, exhale for a count of 5 (no retention or suspension). Repeat 3 times.
- Inhale for a count of 5, hold for a count of 2, exhale for a count of 8, and hold out for a count of 2. Repeat 3 times.
- Inhale for a count of 8, hold for a count of 2, exhale for a count of 10, and hold out for a count of 2. Repeat 3 times.
- Inhale for a count of 5, hold for a count of 2, exhale for a count of 8, and hold out for a count of 2. Repeat 3 times.
- Inhale for a count of 5, exhale for a count of 5 (no retention or suspension). Repeat 3 times.

COOLING BREATH

(Shitali Pranayama)

You probably won't want to perform this breathing exercise in front of a mirror (unless you could use a good laugh). But *Shitali Pranayama* is an effective way to cool the body and calm the mind while expelling toxins from the system. It is also said to relieve a variety of stomach and lower-abdominal ailments. Try this type of breathing on a warm day when the heat has you feeling overwhelmed.

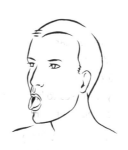

- Sit with your spine comfortably extended.
- Curl the sides of your tongue to form a straw between your lips.
- Inhale through the opening created by your tongue for a count of 7. (Breath count may be modified to suit your comfort level.)
- Withdraw your tongue, close your mouth, and hold your breath for a count of 7.
- Exhale through your nose for a count of 7.
- Repeat 5 or 6 times.

HUMMING BEE BREATH

(Brahmari)

The vibration caused by this exhilarating breath, similar to the one created when chanting *Om*, helps you release tension by calming the body and mind. Focusing on sound and vibration also helps ground you in the present moment, filling you with peace and contentment. As you do this breathing exercise, imagine you are sitting outside on a sunny day, listening to the soothing hum of honeybees working in a flower-filled garden.

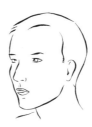

- Sit comfortably with your spine erect.
- Close or lower your eyes.
- Inhale deeply for a count of 7. (Breath count may be modified to suit your comfort level.)
- With lips parted slightly, hum as you exhale for a count of up to 14.
- As the momentum builds, see if you can get your lips to vibrate as you exhale.
- Repeat 2 more times.

SOUNDING BREATH
(*Ujjayi*)

Also known as Victorious Breath, *Ujjayi* is a calming breath that balances the nervous system, slows the mind, and stills the emotions. The sound made by this breath could be compared to that made by the ocean, which can have a tranquilizing influence. You may wish to visualize the cleansing, calming ocean when you practice this type of breathing, which expels stale air from the lungs and purifies the respiratory system.

- Sit with your spine comfortably extended, or lie in Corpse pose (page 127).

- Exhale completely.

- Draw in the breath slowly through your nose, allowing the inhalation to fill your abdomen and lungs.

- Contract the back of your throat slightly and make a soft, hissing sound as you exhale and inhale slowly through the nose. The sound should be audible but not loud, similar to the sound of steam softly escaping from a radiator.

- Continue breathing slowly, focusing on the sound you make, as you inhale and exhale.

- Repeat 3 to 5 times.

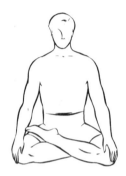

SUCKING BREATH
(*Sitkari Pranayama*)

Many yoga breaths warm and energize, but *Sitkari Pranayama* is also a cooling breath, like *Shitali*, or Cooling Breath (page 27). Because your mouth is open during the inhalation, you may wish not to do this breathing exercise if your teeth and gums are sensitive to the rush of cool air.

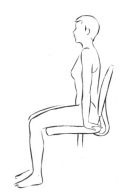

- Place the tip of your tongue on the roof of your mouth just behind your upper teeth.
- With the mouth open but keeping the upper and lower teeth together, draw the breath in through the mouth for a count of 7. (Breath count may be modified to suit your comfort level.)
- Close your mouth and hold for a count of 7.
- Breathe out through your nose for a count of 7.
- Repeat 5 or 6 times.

SUFI MOTHER'S BREATH
(*Sufimata Pranayama*)

Sufi Mother's Breath is said to promote a feeling of safety, security, and nurturing. As with all deep breathing exercises, the increased flow of oxygen improves the complexion and cleanses the inner organs by helping to remove toxins from the system. On the inhalation, concentrate on a sense of well-being that enfolds you like a soft, warm blanket; when you exhale, acknowledge someone in your life who has nurtured and cared for you. Feel protected, secure, and loved.

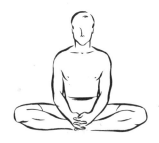

- Sit with your spine comfortably extended, or lie in Corpse pose (page 127).
- Breathe in through the nose for a slow count of 7. Hold the breath in for a count of 1. (Breath count may be modified to suit your comfort level.)
- Breathe out through the nose for a count of 7. Hold the breath out for a count of 1.
- Repeat a few times.

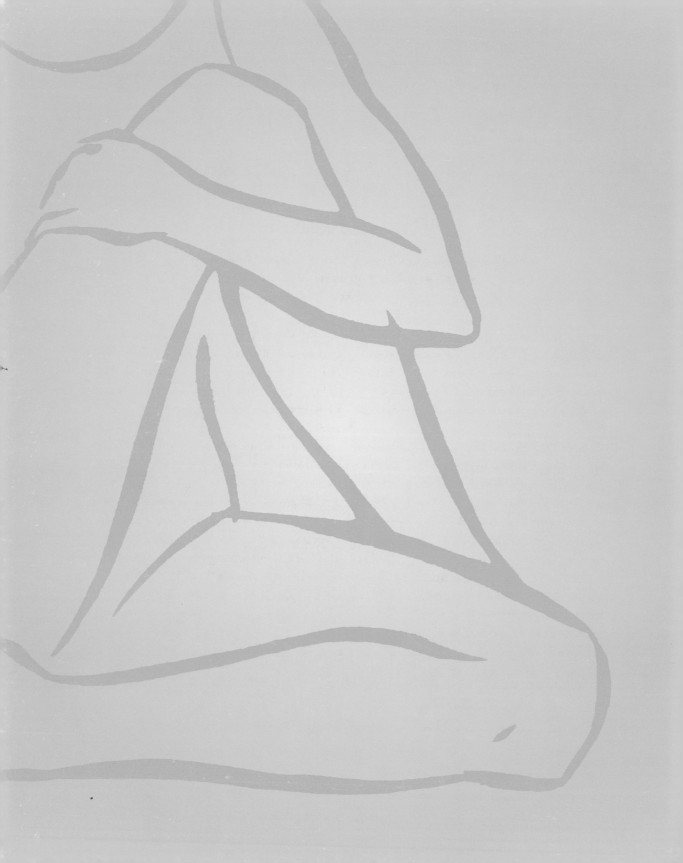

WARM-UPS

TO KEEP THE BODY IN GOOD HEALTH IS A DUTY . . . OTHERWISE WE SHALL NOT
BE ABLE TO KEEP OUR MINDS STRONG AND CLEAR.
—*Buddha*

Admit it: Do you warm up before every yoga workout at home? Or do you usually skip it because you don't have much time . . . or much patience? Your intentions may be good, but next thing you know, you're doing Downward Dog without having stretched your legs first. Bad dog!

I hope this chapter will convince all of us who invariably skip the warm-up that not only is it healthy to warm up before any kind of exercise—including yoga—but it feels good, too. You don't need to make it a long warm-up. Three or four different stretches is all it takes to get the muscles in your neck, shoulders, torso, and legs warmed up and moving. Warming up increases circulation to the parts of your body that you will be using and also helps your mind focus on these areas, resulting in a more effective yoga session.

Warming up for a yoga session is done slowly and with concentration. In general, the warm-ups are simple, dynamic movements that bend, flex, twist, and stretch different parts of the body and prepare you for the more strenuous poses to come. This chapter features 27 warm-ups that can be done standing,

kneeling, sitting, lying on your back, and lying on your stomach. Your body may instinctively let you know which warm-up feels just right, or you may wish to refer to the sessions in chapters 6 and 7 for recommendations on what works best before a particular pose.

One bonus a good warm-up session provides is that you will enjoy similar physical and emotional benefits to those gained from a yoga workout. For example, doing a warm-up such as Knee Hug (page 46) will give your lower back muscles an excellent stretch, massage your entire back and lower abdominal organs, and increase energy throughout your body. A few rounds of Chopping Wood (page 35) will activate and energize the nervous system, work your arms and backs of your legs, and bring a healthy glow to your complexion. And you've reaped these benefits *before* you've actually started your yoga session.

I hope you're convinced that the warm-up is an integral part of a yoga practice. But don't take my word for it. Try a few of the following warm-ups and experience the benefits for yourself.

STANDING PELVIC TILT

(*Paryutthita Vastinirvlina*)

You can do Standing Pelvic Tilt almost anywhere or anytime—at work or while waiting in line (you don't really need a wall to lean against; simply tilt your pelvis as you stand). This warm-up helps prevent and relieve lower back fatigue, strengthens the abdominal muscles, and promotes an overall feeling of relaxation.

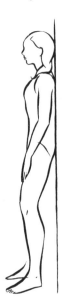

- Stand with your back against a wall. Your heels should be about 6 inches from the wall.

- Keep your feet separated and parallel and your knees slightly bent. You can rest your hands on your thighs, by your sides, or along the wall.

- On an exhalation, tilt your pubic bone up and tailbone down by contracting your abdominal muscles. Inhale as your lower back presses against the wall.

- Repeat this subtle pelvic movement several times.

BARREL MOVEMENT
(*Kabandha*)

Loosen your back and hips as you move your lower body in a circular motion, as if you were using a hoola hoop. This slow, hypnotic movement increases flexibility in the lower back, loosens the hips, relaxes the body, and calms the mind.

- Stand with your feet about hip-distance apart. Arms hang loosely by your sides. Make sure your spine is comfortably extended, your shoulders are down away from your ears, and your abdominal muscles are slightly engaged.

- Close or lower your eyes.

FIG. 1:

- Inhale and slowly begin making small circles with your hips in a clockwise direction.

- Gradually allow the circles to expand so that your hips are moving in large circles. Try to keep your upper body stationary; the movement should be in your hips only. Imagine that you've wrapped a towel around your hips and that you are trying to clean the inside of a barrel.

- Continue for 12 clockwise circles.

- Stop. Breathe and feel the energy swirling in your hips, lower back, and abdomen.

FIG. 2:

- Resume by making small circles in the opposite (counterclockwise) direction.

- Gradually increase the size of your circles. Make the inside of that barrel shine!

- Make 12 circles. Stop. Relax as you enjoy feeling the energy whirl.

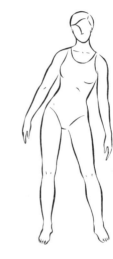

FIG. 1

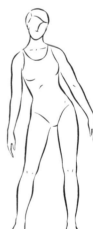

FIG. 2

TORSO TWIST
(Madhyadeha Parivrttana)

We used to do this when we were kids, just for the fun of it. As a warm-up, it loosens up your arms, torso, spine, and waist. Try it anytime you realize you've been sitting too long and haven't moved around much. It will energize your upper body and make you feel like a little kid again.

- Stand with your feet about shoulder-width apart. Your spine is comfortably extended, and your shoulders are away from the ears. Your arms hang loosely by your sides.

- Engage your abdominal muscles slightly.

FIG. 1:

- Begin turning your upper body, shoulder first, from one side to the other. As you alternate, allow your arms to swing slowly as though they were empty coat sleeves.

- Let your head follow the movement of your upper body.

FIG. 2:

- As you pick up the pace, allow the heel of your right foot to come off the floor when your body turns to the left. Your left heel rises when your body turns to the right.

- Repeat this side-to-side motion for as long as you like.

- When you feel ready, slow the motion and gradually return to center. Feel the energy stream through your body.

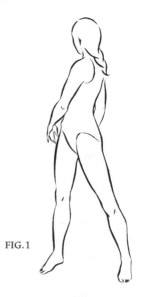

FIG. 1

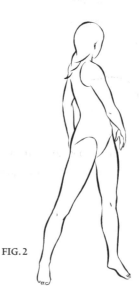

FIG. 2

CHOPPING WOOD
(Kashtha Cchindana)

This warm-up is guaranteed to awaken your whole system and get things moving by increasing your heart rate and respiration. The circulation throughout your body will increase, and your complexion will improve. The easy forward-bending motion limbers up your back and lessens neck strain. Don't perform this warm-up if you have high blood pressure, heart disease, or glaucoma.

• Stand with legs about shoulder-width apart. Keep your knees slightly bent to avoid strain in the lower back.

FIG. 1:

• Inhale through your mouth and raise your arms over your head as if you were holding a hatchet.

FIG. 2:

• Bend your knees. Exhale through your mouth, slightly tuck your chin, and bend from the waist while allowing your arms to fall forward and down in a chopping motion. Bend as far as you can with comfort.

• Inhale and raise your upper body.

• Continue this "chopping" movement 12 times. Increase the flow of energy by making each exhalation audible. As you repeat the movement, your body may naturally bend further as your arms get closer to the floor. If it feels comfortable, allow the natural swing of your arms to go through your legs.

• Return to a standing position and lower your arms. Feel the energy course through your body.

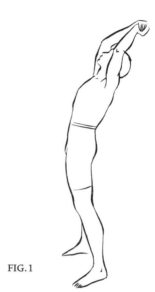

FIG. 1

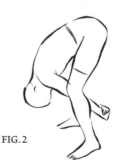

FIG. 2

WATER WHEEL
(Vaari Chakrasana)

This dynamic warm-up releases tension in the pelvic area, limbers the spinal column, and increases respiration and circulation while energizing the entire system. Imagine the energy moving up and down your spine in a smooth, fluid motion, like water cascading over a dam. Don't perform this warm-up if you have high blood pressure, heart disease, or glaucoma.

- Stand with your feet about shoulder-width apart, with knees slightly bent.

FIG. 1:

- Place your palms against your lower back, fingers pointing down.

- Relax your lower jaw as you open your mouth slightly. Inhale through the mouth and arch backward, gently pressing your hands into your lower back for support. Gaze upward, keeping your neck in line with the spine to avoid putting any pressure on your neck.

FIG. 2:

- Exhale through the mouth and "spill" forward like a water wheel, bringing your chin toward your chest and letting your upper body hang and arms dangle. Keep your knees bent.

- Repeat the movement 8 to 12 times. Feel free to add sound when you exhale to really get your energy flowing.

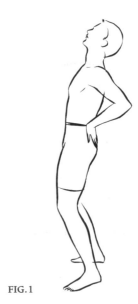

FIG. 1

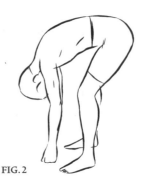

FIG. 2

HANDS-TO-WALL STRETCH

(*Kudya Hastya*)

This movement tones and strengthens the muscles of the upper chest and strengthens the arms and wrists. The farther you stand from the wall, the more energetic the exercise will be and the more you will work your chest and arm muscles.

FIG. 1:

- Stand with your spine comfortably extended, arms shoulder-distance apart in front of you with your palms against the wall.

- Position your body so you are an arm's length from the wall. Your body is straight, leaning in at a slight angle.

- The fingers of both hands point toward each other slightly, touching but not overlapping. (If this is uncomfortable, adjust the hand position.) Your shoulders are relaxed, and your feet are flat on the floor. Engage the abdominals to prevent arching in the lower back.

FIG. 2:

- Inhale. Exhale and slowly bend the elbows so that, gradually and with control, your upper body moves toward the wall.

- Bring your face as close to the wall as you can with comfort. Your body remains straight. Do not bend at the waist or knees.

- Hold for a few moments, breathing normally.

- Inhale and slowly push away from the wall until your arms are straight and your body is erect. Lower your arms. Relax and breathe normally.

- Repeat 8 to 10 times.

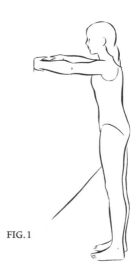

FIG. 1

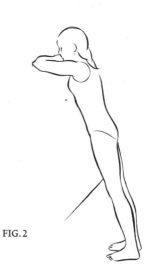

FIG. 2

CAT AND DOG STRETCH

(*Bidala Kukkuta Uttana*)

As you alternate between an angry hunchback cat and a happy swayback dog, you increase the suppleness of your spine; stretch the muscles along your back, neck, and arms; and improve circulation. Doing Cat and Dog Stretch will keep your spine flexible and strong, so important to maintaining good posture and overall well-being.

- Kneel in "table position," with knees under hips and arms beneath the shoulders.
- Your back is flat, and your head faces downward to create an extension in the back of the neck.

FIG. 1:

- Exhale and slowly drop your head and tailbone. Arch your back and exhale further as you pull your navel up toward your spine. Imagine you are a hissing cat.

FIG. 2:

- Inhale and slowly raise your head and tailbone, letting your abdomen move toward the floor. Your back is now curved in a subtle swayback position. Look up slightly without overextending the neck. Imagine you are a friendly dog.
- Continue alternating, moving slowly between cat and dog 10 times.
- As your spine warms up, deepen your inhalations and exhalations.

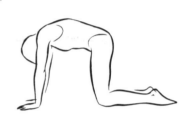

FIG. 1

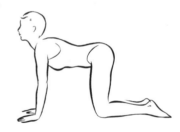

FIG. 2

SIDE-TO-SIDE STRETCH

(*Anyonya Paksa Nayana*)

Here's a wonderful warm-up that perhaps you've never done—moving your spine from one side to the other as though you were a dog trying to see its own tail by looking to one side, then the other. This side-to-side movement also keeps the spine flexible and stretches the muscles along the sides of the upper torso. Do this after Cat and Dog Stretch (facing page), which moves the spine in a different direction; done together, these two stretches will greatly reduce any stiffness caused by too much sitting and inactivity.

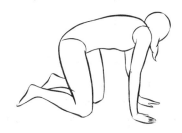

- Kneel in "table position," with knees under hips and arms beneath the shoulders.

- Your back is straight, and your head faces downward.

- Turn your head to the left so that you are looking behind you. At the same time, move your lower body to the left so that your body is in the shape of a comma. Don't strain. Feel a gentle stretch on the right side of the body.

- Now reverse the stretch so you are making a comma of your body on the right side. Feel a gentle stretch on the left side of your body.

- Alternate 5 times on each side.

THREADING THE NEEDLE

(*Suci Sutrana*)

Feel tension dissipate after a few rounds of Threading the Needle. This warm-up loosens the muscles in the back, shoulders, and neck while releasing tension in the neck and shoulders. At the same time, it massages the abdominal organs and relaxes and refreshes the entire system.

- Begin in "table position," with arms under shoulders and knees under hips.
- Imagine that your right hand holds a needle and long thread. Inhale and lift your right arm out to the side and then up toward the ceiling; if your neck permits, allow your gaze to follow your hand.

FIG. 1:

- Exhale and thread the imaginary needle through the space under your left arm. Allow your right shoulder, upper arm, and side of the face to "melt" into the floor.
- Remain in this position for several seconds. Let your breath help you soften further into the pose.

FIG. 2:

- For an added stretch, raise your left arm toward the ceiling. If your neck feels okay, look up at your raised hand.
- Make small, slow clockwise circles, gradually increasing in size; then reverse direction.
- Slowly return to "table position" and repeat on other side.

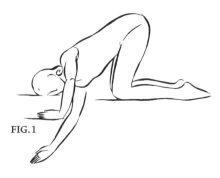

FIG. 1

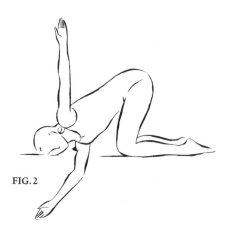

FIG. 2

NECK ROLLS
(*Kantha Luthana*)

Most of us find that our necks bear the brunt of the stress and tension in our lives. These simple neck movements can be done while you're sitting at your desk, watching television, or waiting for the train. One side of your neck may be tighter than the other, so be gentle and don't overstretch. The popping or gritting noises you may hear will usually subside over time. The movements lubricate and stretch the neck joints and relieve residual tension in the neck and shoulders.

- Sit with your spine comfortably extended and your head upright.

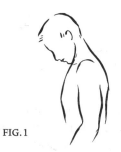

FIG. 1

FIG. 1:

- Exhale and drop your head forward, with your chin toward your chest.

- Inhale and raise your head up so that chin is level with the floor.

- Repeat 5 to 7 times.

FIG. 2:

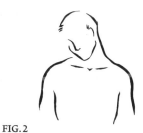

FIG. 2

- With your head upright, slowly drop your left ear toward your left shoulder. Hold for a few breaths, allowing the right side of your neck to release.

- Let your right hand fall toward the floor and allow it to pull your right shoulder down slightly to *gently* increase the stretch.

- Take your left hand and place it just above your right ear. Increase the stretch by adding some *gentle* pressure with your hand, increasing the stretch ever so slightly. Be careful not to tug or pull your head to the left. Hold for 8 to 10 seconds.

- Relax the left hand to the floor, returning your head to an upright position.

- Perform the stretch on the opposite side.

SHOULDER SHRUGS, CIRCLES, AND TWISTS

(*Amsha Vrttana, Amsha Cakra, Amsha Parivrttana*)

If there's one place where we hold tension, it is usually the neck and shoulders. The next time you feel tense (during a difficult meeting, while waiting for an important phone call, after a trying day), notice if your neck aches and your shoulders are hunched up and tight. These three movements will cure what ails you while improving flexibility in the upper back, shoulders, and arms; stretching the muscles along the upper torso; and increasing upper arm strength.

- Sit in a comfortable position.

FIG. 1:

- Bring both shoulders up toward the ears as high as you can. Exaggerate the shrug and accentuate the holding.

- Release, letting shoulders drop back and down.

- Repeat a few times.

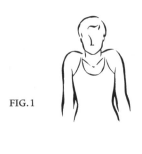

FIG. 1

FIG. 2:

- Bend both elbows and lightly place your fingertips on top of your shoulders.

- Rotate your elbows as though you were drawing small circles on the walls.

- Circle 5 times in one direction; reverse direction and circle 5 more times.

- Drop your arms. As you breathe deeply, focus on how relaxed your neck and shoulders feel.

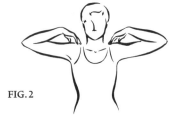

FIG. 2

FIG. 3:

- Once again, bend both elbows and lightly place your hands on your shoulders.

- Inhale and exhale while, slowly and with control, turn your upper torso and head to the right. Hold for a few seconds.

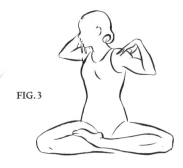

FIG. 3

- Inhale and return to center. Exhale and slowly turn your upper torso and head to the left. Hold for a few seconds.

- Inhale and return to center. Repeat 8 to 10 times on each side. Without straining or forcing, engage the abdominal muscles slightly (to support the back) and try to turn a bit further each time.

BLADE

(Kshura Asana)

This warm-up not only feels good, but it can be done at your desk whenever you need a quick refresher. It helps tone and strengthen the pectoral muscles and opens the chest. The Blade also releases tension held between the shoulder blades, helping to relax the entire body.

- Sit in a comfortable position with your spine extended.

FIG. 1:

- Inhale, raising your arms out to the sides at shoulder level in a T position. Bend your elbows so your arms are in front of your chest, palms down. Your hands come toward each other with the tips of the middle fingers touching lightly.

FIG. 2:

- Exhale. Inhale slowly as you gradually push backward with your elbows so that your hands move away from one another. Feel your shoulder blades come together with a steady, squeezing motion.

- Hold the position, with your arms as far back as is comfortable, for a few seconds, breathing normally.

- Exhale and, with focus, bring your arms back to start position.

- Repeat the movement slowly 3 to 5 times.

- Exhale and gradually release the position, letting your arms fall to your sides. Relax by shrugging your shoulders and gently shaking out your hands a few times.

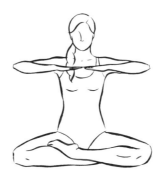

FIG. 1

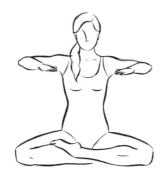

FIG. 2

FULL BODY STRETCH

(*Sarva Kaya Uttana*)

Do this warm-up before your yoga session to make sure your body is completely stretched out and ready for the upcoming poses. It loosens up the muscles of your arms, legs, and torso while stretching your spinal column to its fullest length. Coordinating your breath with the movement removes toxins and increases circulation throughout the body. This is also a great stretch to do in bed when you wake up in the morning.

- Lie on your back. Make sure your chin is not higher than your forehead. If you feel any strain in your neck, place a folded blanket or towel under your head.

- On an inhalation, bring your arms up over your head and onto the floor so that the backs of your hands rest on the mat or towel. Be careful not to overstretch your shoulder joints.

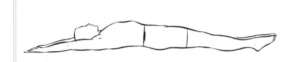

- Exhale and stretch your arms and legs in opposite directions. Open your hands so the fingers are splayed; point your toes. Open your mouth and your eyes wide.

- Really *stretch*.

- Imagine that a friend has taken hold of your wrists while another friend holds your ankles. Together they gently and lovingly pull on your wrists and ankles, giving you the best stretch you've ever had.

- Continue to breathe, stretching further with each exhalation.

- Exhale deeply, return your arms to your sides, and relax your entire body. Feel a sense of letting go as you release further into the floor.

KNEE DOWN TWIST

(Adho Janunah Parivrtta Asana)

This exercise will warm up your back and hips. It's a great stretch to do before Pigeon (page 117).

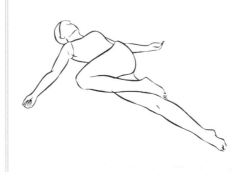

- Lie on your back with legs extended and about hip-distance apart. Make sure your chin is not higher than your forehead. If you feel any strain in your neck, place a folded blanket or towel under your head.

- Extend your arms out to each side in a T position, palms turned up.

- Bend your left knee. Place the left foot lightly on the right thigh wherever it is comfortable.

- Try to keep your left shoulder on the floor. Inhale.

- On an exhalation, begin to lower your left knee to the right so that it crosses over your body.

- To assist in lowering your knee to the floor, place your right hand on your left knee and use it to *gently* and *gradually* guide your knee to the right.

- Do not let your left hip go beyond the imaginary vertical line formed by both hips. Your left hip may be stacked above the right, but don't allow it to go any further.

- If your neck permits, slowly turn your head to the left without straining.

- Breathe deeply as you hold the twist for 15 to 30 seconds.

- Inhale and return your left leg to the center. Feel the results.

- Straighten the leg and complete the posture on the other side. Compare your right and left hips and notice the differences.

- Repeat a few times on each side.

KNEE HUG

(Apanasana)

Can't get thee to a massage therapist? Treat yourself to a simple and effective lower back massage with Knee Hug. This warm-up stretches the lower back muscles while massaging the entire back and the lower abdominal organs. Feel energy being restored to your entire body.

- Lie on your back with your head resting comfortably on the floor. Make sure your chin is not higher than your forehead. If you feel any strain in your neck, place a folded blanket or towel under your head.

- Bend both knees and bring them to your chest.

- Wrap your arms around both shins, grasping your forearms or wrists. Lightly squeeze your legs.

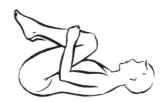

- Gently roll from side to side, massaging the lower back. Your head rests comfortably on the floor and moves in the same direction as the body.

- For a variation, unfold your arms and place your hands on your knees. Part your knees slightly and make slow circles with them, massaging your hips and sacrum into the floor.

- Allow your movements to be slow and gentle. Your head stays on the floor at all times.

ALTERNATING KNEE HUG

(Apanasana II)

This warm-up provides the same benefits as Knee Hug but is more energetic, since it tones the abdominal muscles. In addition, it strengthens the neck muscles, which can gradually weaken as we grow older. It also helps restore energy throughout the body. Alternating Knee Hug is a great stretch to do after a long day at the office.

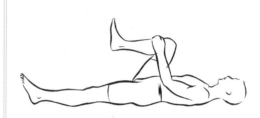

- Lie on your back. Make sure your chin is not higher than your forehead. If you feel any strain in your neck, place a folded blanket or towel under your head.

- Bring both knees into your chest. If your neck permits, raise your forehead to your knees, keeping space between your chin and chest. Keep your shoulders down and away from your ears throughout the repetitions. If you experience discomfort in your neck, lower your head back down to the floor.

- Interlace your fingers below your right knee. Exhale and extend your left leg forward and press your lower back into the floor, keeping the entire leg about 8 inches off the floor.

- Inhale and bring your left knee back into the chest.

- Interlace your fingers below your left knee. Exhale and extend your right leg forward and press your lower back into the floor, keeping the entire right leg about 8 inches off the floor.

- Make sure your lower back stays flat on the floor. Do not allow it to arch or lift.

- Alternate slowly for 10 to 12 repetitions.

TRUNK ROTATIONS

(Madhyadeha Vrttana)

This warm-up will help keep your spine flexible while stretching your neck and shoulders. It tones the waistline and strengthens the abdominals and the muscles along the torso. Do this whenever your upper body and neck could use a good stretch.

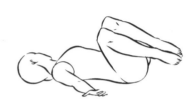

- Lie on your back with legs extended about hip-distance apart. Make sure your chin is not higher than your forehead. If you feel any strain in your neck, place a folded blanket or towel under your head.

- Bend your legs and bring both knees to your chest.

- Extend your arms to each side in a T position, palms turned up.

- Inhale. On an exhalation, bring your legs 3 to 5 inches to the right, while turning your head slowly to the left. Keep your legs close together. Don't allow the sides of your legs to touch the floor. Keep your abdominal muscles and the muscles along the sides of your body engaged.

- Inhale and use your inhalation to help raise your knees and head back to center. Exhale in a controlled manner, and let your knees go to the right, while your head turns to the left. Again, don't let your legs touch the floor.

- Alternate sides 8 to 10 times.

TRUNK ROTATIONS WITH RAISED ARMS

(*Uditabahu Madhyadeha Vrttana*)

This twist is a bit more challenging than Trunk Rotations. Although your legs won't be able to drop as close to the floor, this is a great workout for the abdominal muscles. It also massages the internal organs.

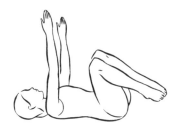

- Follow the first two bullets in the instructions for Trunk Rotations.
- Lift your arms off the floor and raise them parallel to each other with fingertips pointing to the ceiling. Now try moving your bent legs to one side as you turn your head in the opposite direction.

SPINAL ROCKING

(*Prstha Ashti*)

This is a good preparation for the Half Shoulderstand (page 130), Full Shoulderstand (page 131), and Plough (page 132). This warm-up strengthens the abdominal muscles and stretches the back muscles. Do not do this pose if you have a herniated disc.

FIG. 1:

- Lying on your back, bring your knees into your chest and place your hands beneath the knees. Slowly bring your forehead toward your knees.
- From this position, begin to rock 2 to 3 inches forward and back, massaging your spine.

FIG. 2:

- If your spine is flexible enough, inhale and rock up onto your sitting bones. Exhale, keep your chin toward the chest, leaving space between the chin and chest, and rock back *only* onto your upper back and shoulders, *not* onto your neck or head.
- Continue rocking for 4 to 6 breaths.

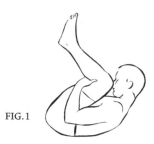

FIG. 1

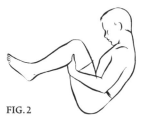

FIG. 2

LEG LIFTS

(Nalaka Udayana)

This warm-up engages and strengthens the muscles of the leg. Make sure your upper body is relaxed and that there is no strain on your neck or back.

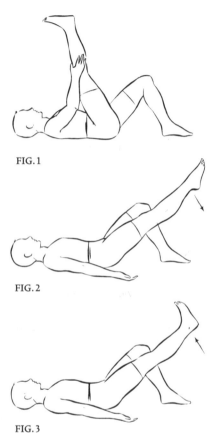

FIG. 1

FIG. 2

FIG. 3

- Lie on your back with both legs extended on the floor. Make sure your chin is not higher than your forehead. If you feel any strain in your neck, place a folded blanket or towel under your head.

- Bend your left leg, ensuring that your lower back does not arch.

FIG. 1:

- Inhale and lift your straight right leg, with the bottom of the foot parallel to the ceiling, as far as you comfortably can.

- Using both hands, vigorously massage the hamstring muscle at the back of your thigh for about 10 seconds.

- Lower your hands to the calf muscle and *gently* pull back on the leg. Use a strap or tie if you are unable to reach comfortably. Do not allow your hip or buttock to lift off the floor.

FIG. 2:

- Release the leg. Exhale and slowly begin to lower your straight leg. Point your toes as you lower the leg to within a few inches from the floor.

FIG. 3:

- Just before your heel touches the floor, inhale and flex the toes toward the ceiling as you slowly raise the leg back up. Continue 8 to 10 times with the same leg, pointing the toes as you lower your leg and flexing the toes as you raise it back up.

- On the last repetition, lower your leg to a few inches from the floor, flex your toes back toward the shin, press out through the heel, and lightly touch the top of your thigh with your fingers.

- Lower your leg. Now straighten both legs on the floor and compare how they feel. Notice the difference between them.

- Repeat with the opposite leg.

ALTERNATING LEG LIFTS

(Prthak Nalaka Udayana)

Remember that in this warm-up, it doesn't matter how far you lower your legs. What is important is that your lower back remains flat on the floor. If your back starts to arch as you lower your leg, stop at that angle and raise your leg back to vertical. This warm-up works the abdominal muscles and strengthens the neck muscles. It also strengthens and increases flexibility of the thigh muscles. This is an energizing warm-up that is good to do before any exercises that use the lower extremities.

- Lie on your back with both legs extended on the floor. Make sure your chin is not higher than your forehead. If you feel any strain in your neck, place a folded blanket or towel under your head.

FIG. 1:

- Bring both knees to your chest.

- Engage your abdominal muscles 20 percent by pulling your navel toward your spine. Keep the lower back in contact with the floor. Do not arch it.

- Exhale and lower your toes to the floor approximately 12 inches from your buttocks. Inhale and bring your knees back up to your chest.

- Do 8 to 10 repetitions.

FIG. 2:

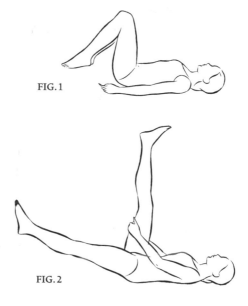

FIG. 1

FIG. 2

- For a more challenging warm-up, extend both legs up vertically. Your legs may be at an angle less than 90° if your hamstrings are tight.

- If your neck permits, raise your forehead toward your knees. Keep your shoulders down and away from your ears. Allow space between your chin and chest.

- Place both hands behind your right leg. Exhale and lower the left leg toward the floor without arching your lower back.

- Inhale and raise your left leg back up. Place both hands behind it. Exhale and lower the right leg toward the floor without arching your lower back.

- Alternate on each side 6 to 10 times, creating a scissor-like movement.

LEG STRETCH

(*Nalaka Uttana*)

It is important to maintain suppleness as we age. Do this stretch regularly and watch your flexibility improve. This warm-up stretches the muscles and tendons along the back of the legs and prepares the lower body for more strenuous stretches. Runners, bicyclists, dancers, and people who walk a lot should be sure to incorporate this stretch into their regular routine.

- Lie on your back with your legs bent, feet flat on the floor. Make sure your chin is not higher than your forehead. If you feel any strain in your neck, place a folded blanket or towel under your head.

FIG. 1:

- Raise your left leg to a vertical position. With both hands, grasp behind your leg wherever you can reach *comfortably,* either ankle or calf.

- Gently pull your leg toward your chest. *Don't strain*.

FIG. 2:

- To help increase the stretch, bend your leg and loop a tie or scarf over the sole of your foot. Grab the tie so that both your elbows are straight. Straighten your leg and *gently* pull on the ends of the tie, bringing the leg toward the chest.

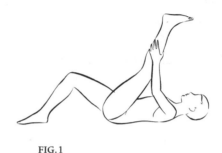

FIG. 1

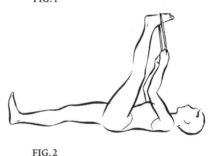

FIG. 2

- With each exhalation, allow your leg to come closer to your chest. Don't force the stretch . . . you'll only end up with sore muscles.

- If your lower back feels comfortable and remains flat on the floor, straighten the other leg.

- Hold for several relaxed breaths.

- Repeat with the opposite leg.

PELVIC TILT

(Vasti Nirvlina)

This is a great way to prepare your back for Bridge pose (page 120). It loosens up the lower back, relieves any back strain or tension, and strengthens the abdominal muscles. It's also a great warm-up to do simply because it feels great.

- Lie on your back with hands on abdomen or with arms a comfortable distance from the body, with palms up.

- Make sure your chin is not higher than your forehead. If you feel any strain in your neck, place a folded blanket or towel under your head.

- Legs are separated about hip-distance apart, with insteps parallel. Knees are bent to help lengthen the lower back.

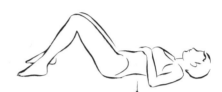

- On an exhalation, pull the navel toward the spine. Abdominal muscles are contracted.

- Inhale and relax the abdominal muscles; on the exhalation, continue to pull your navel toward the spine.

- Feel increased circulation in the lower back and a lengthening of the lumbar (lower) spine as though your tailbone were lengthening toward the front of the room. The buttocks stay on the floor at all times.

- Repeat 8 to 10 times.

PELVIC LIFT

(*Vasti Udayana*)

This warm-up starts out like Pelvic Tilt (page 53), but eventually you lift your pelvis off the floor. It is also an excellent preparation for Bridge pose (page 120), a strenuous posture that shouldn't be done before warming up the back first. Pelvic Lift also works the legs and buttock muscles.

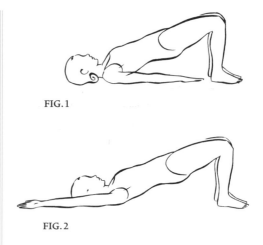

FIG. 1

FIG. 2

- Lie on your back with your arms a comfortable distance from the body, with palms down.

- Make sure your chin is not higher than your forehead. If you feel any strain in your neck, place a folded blanket or towel under your head.

- Your legs should be separated about hip-distance apart, with insteps parallel. Your knees are bent to help lengthen the lower back.

- Maintain a slight pelvic tilt.

FIG. 1:

- On an inhalation, press evenly into the soles of the feet and raise your pelvis an inch from the floor. Exhale the pelvis down to the floor.

- Inhale, press into the soles of your feet, and raise your pelvis 2 inches from the floor. We often have a tendency to externally rotate our legs and feet. Don't put all your weight on the outside of your feet—make sure there is an even distribution of weight at the soles of your feet. Feel your big toes and inner heel mounds pressing down.

- With each inhalation, gradually begin to lift the pelvis a little higher. Use your inhalations and exhalations to smoothly lift and lower the tailbone, sacrum, lower back, and possibly part of your thoracic spine (between the neck and abdomen) off the floor. Listen to your body to determine a comfortable elevation.

FIG. 2:

- For a variation, inhale and press into the soles of the feet. If it feels okay, simultaneously raise your pelvis and both arms over your head and onto the floor—if the shoulders permit. The backs of your hands are on the floor. Honor any limitations in your shoulders.

- Return your arms to your sides as you exhale and lower the pelvis.

- Repeat this movement a few more times, raising the pelvis as high as you comfortably can.

- When you're ready, bring your knees to the chest, wrapping your arms below the knees in Knee Hug (page 46), a great counterpose.

SUPINE BUTTERFLY

(Urdhva Shayana Patamgama)

Those who are already flexible in the hips and upper thighs will relish the openings that Supine Butterfly creates; those who are tighter in this area will find that this warm-up eventually improves flexibility. Don't force this exercise. Breathe into any areas of tightness and allow your legs to fall open a bit more with each exhalation. By creating resistance with your hands as your legs return to center, you'll also strengthen your inner thigh and arm muscles. It also brings extra blood to the pelvic floor and is beneficial to the reproductive glands.

FIG. 1:

- Lie on your back with knees bent and your feet flat on the floor. Make sure your chin is not higher than your forehead. If you feel any strain in your neck, place a folded blanket or towel under your head.

- Bring the soles of your feet together and allow your knees to splay out to each side.

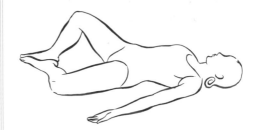

FIG. 1

FIG. 2:

- Inhale and slowly begin to bring your knees back up toward each other. As they return to center, press your hands into your inner thighs to create resistance.

- Make it a leisurely journey of up to 45 seconds before your knees meet again. Repeat twice more.

- While on your back extend both legs up vertically, placing your hands on the inner thighs.

- Inhale and separate your legs as far as is comfortable.

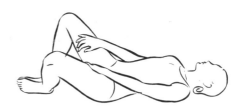

FIG. 2

- Exhale and bring your legs back to vertical, pressing your hands into the inner thighs, creating resistance. Continue this movement for 5 to 7 repetitions. Listen to your breath as you perform the repetitions.

- Give yourself permission to make any sounds as you do this movement.

SPHINX

It is important to do whatever we can to keep our backs flexible and strong. This warm-up contracts and strengthens the lower back muscles and stretches the abdominal muscles.

- Lie on your stomach, with legs hip-distance apart.
- Raise your head and chest as you prop yourself up onto your bent elbows. Your forearms are flat on the floor, shoulder width apart, with palms facing down.
- Let your pelvis lean toward the floor by engaging your abdominal muscles 15 to 20 percent. Your head and neck remain neutral.
- Breathe and hold for a count of 10.
- Lower and repeat 3 to 5 times.

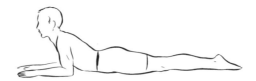

WINDSHIELD WIPER LEGS

You might remember doing something like this warm-up when you were a kid watching television. It gets your legs moving and keeps the lower body flexible. It is also an effective counterpose to Cobra (page 111) and Bow (page 113).

- Lie on your stomach. Your head may be turned to one side, or your chin can rest on top of your hands.
- Legs are about hip-distance apart.
- Bend the legs at the knees.

FIGS. 1 & 2:

- Slowly move both legs from one side to the other in a "windshield wiper" movement.
- Continue this movement several times and feel your lower back relax.

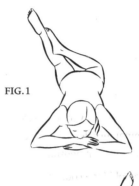

FIG. 1

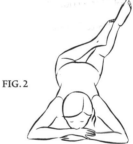

FIG. 2

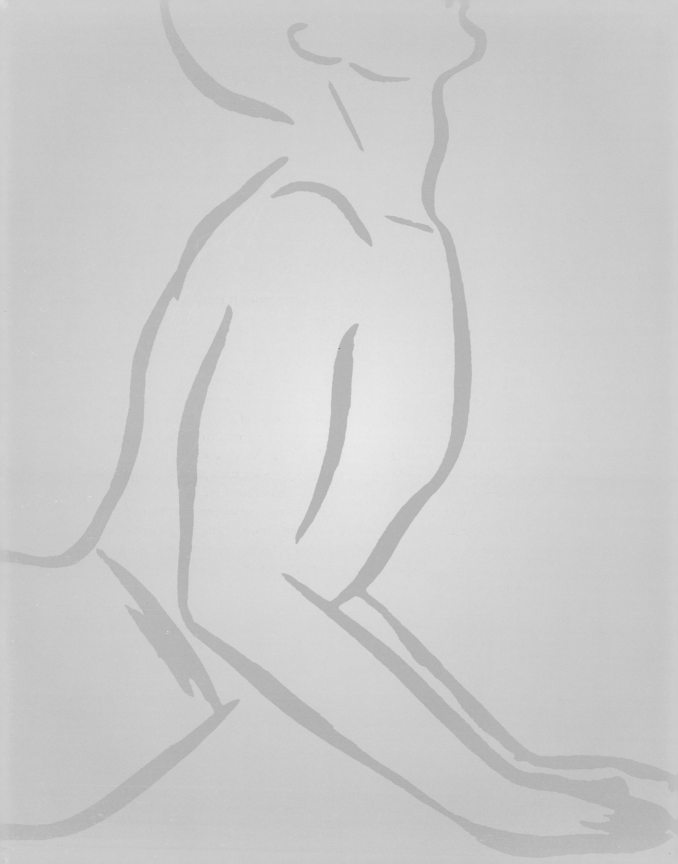

3

YOGA POSES

THE GREATER THE EMPHASIS ON PERFECTION, THE FURTHER IT RECEDES.
—Haridas Chaudhuri

As you begin your yoga session, try to enter into your practice with a sense of *maitri*, a Sanskrit word that translates as "unconditional friendliness toward one's own experience." This is quite different from striving to be what you *think* you should be—an idealized version of yourself—the one without the stiff knees, tight hamstrings, or sore neck. Once you think you should be different from what you are, you become disconnected from the experience, which greatly diminishes your yoga practice.

If, instead, you give yourself permission to be who you are, if you open up and relax into *maitri*, a softening and unfolding can occur—from the inside out. We can practice *maitri* when we're off the mat as well. As you go about your day, express an attitude of openness, awareness, and acceptance toward yourself, your experiences, and others.

Remember that *asana*, the Sanskrit word for pose, means "posture comfortably held." You are not out to "feel the burn." Try to hold the pose to the edge of your tolerance. Don't force yourself beyond this limit. Allow your breath, not competitiveness or ego, to fuel and energize your body. If your muscles are tight, direct the breath to that area. Go to where you feel the stretch and hold it at that point; inhale deeply, and on an exhalation, see if you can deepen into the stretch. Try repeating the pose. The first time, your body and mind may not be prepared; the second time, you know what's expected so you may have a very different experience.

Use this time to focus inward. If you practice the poses in a quiet space and attend to what is happening moment to moment, you are actually practicing a form of meditation in motion. Don't rush, don't strive, don't overdo it. Be aware and be yourself.

This section focuses on poses done from a standing position. These dynamic poses energize, stretch, and strengthen your body as well as increase your focus and concentration. When you prepare for a pose, make sure your body is aligned and your spine is comfortably extended. Allow the skeletal system to support the body. For example, in Mountain pose (see below), sense that your ears are over your shoulders, shoulders positioned over your hips, hips over ankles. Stand as though you have grown an inch. Pull your shoulders back slightly, down and away from your ears. Splay your toes and press them into the floor.

In poses where you are bent over, soften your knees if your muscles feel tight and tuck your chin slightly toward your chest; when coming back up, roll your body up slowly, keeping your knees soft and chin slightly lifted so your head comes up last. If balancing poses present a challenge, hold onto a wall or the back of a chair. Gaze at a spot in front of you and breathe deeply; with practice, your balance will improve.

MOUNTAIN
(*Tadasana*)

Mountain is a fundamental pose that provides the proper alignment for other standing poses. It helps correct any posture problems we may have developed, while restoring a natural state of balance to the body and mind. (You may also want to try Seated Mountain, page 92.)

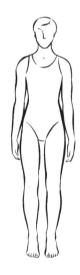

- Stand erect, with legs hip-width apart and feet parallel. Place half of your weight onto your heels, the other half onto the balls of your feet. Feel your big toes pressing down.

- Allow your thighbones to move toward your hamstring muscles in the back of your legs. Feel your kneecaps lift.

- Feel yourself lifting out of your waist. Your shoulders are relaxed and down, and your chin is level with the floor. Retract your chin slightly to feel a lengthening in the back of your neck.

- Inhale deeply, filling the lungs. Keep your arms by your sides or raise them overhead with palms facing each other. Relax your shoulders as you stretch from the armpits.

- Gaze ahead; hold for 8 to 10 breaths. If your arms are raised, release them and let them slowly float down to your sides.

STANDING-ON-TOES

(Prapada Sthana)

In addition to strengthening the calf muscles, this pose stretches the soles of the feet, massages the balls of the feet, helps with balance, and increases concentration.

- Stand in Mountain pose (facing page), with arms by your sides.

FIG. 1:

- Inhale and raise your heels from the floor, rising up onto the balls of your feet. Exhale and come back down.

- Repeat this up and down movement for 4 to 6 breaths.

FIG. 2:

- Inhale and lift your heels from the floor, rising up onto the balls of your feet and raising your arms overhead.

- Repeat this up and down movement with your feet and arms several times.

- Remain on your toes with the arms raised for 4 to 6 breaths.

- Return your feet to the floor and your arms to your sides.

- Repeat once more.

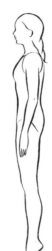

FIG. 1

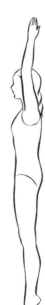

FIG. 2

HALF MOON
(*Ardha Chandrasana*)

Half Moon bends your body so that it resembles a crescent moon. As your body bends first to one side and then to the other, it reinforces how supple and flexible your entire being is. If you do both rounds of Half Moon, you'll likely stretch further the second time. This deceptively simple pose stretches the muscles at the waist and along the sides of the upper body, and trims and tones the waistline. It also stretches the arms and aligns the spine. (You may also wish to try Seated Half Moon, page 92.)

- Stand with your feet parallel and close together.

- Raise both arms overhead, palms facing each other. If it feels comfortable, cross your thumbs.

- Tighten your thigh muscles to feel a lifting of the kneecaps.

- Create an extension in your spine and slowly and gently bend out of the waist to the left.

- Angle your upper body slightly to the left and look down at your left foot. Make sure there is no strain in your neck.

- Hold for a few breaths.

- Return your upper body to the center. If your shoulders have inched up, drop them down away from the ears.

- Repeat on the right side. Don't strain. Hold for several breaths.

- Return to center. Relax your arms.

- Repeat once more on both sides.

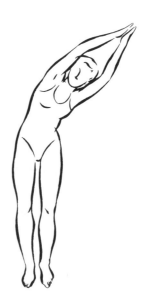

TRIANGLE
(Trikonasana)

A triangle is a geometric form that embodies strength, balance, and support. This ancient posture, which replicates the innate stability of a triangle, improves flexibility of the torso, elongates and straightens the spine, opens the hip area, and strengthens the arms, legs, ankles, and feet. Concentrate on holding the pose in stillness while you breathe deeply and rhythmically. Feel the solidity and strength of the triangle fill your entire being and rest firmly in the knowledge that nothing can shake the solid foundation that is your core.

- Stand with your feet separated about 3 feet apart or the length of one leg.
- Turn your right foot out 90°; turn your left foot in (toward the right) about 30°.

FIG. 1:

- As you inhale, stretch your arms out from your shoulders so they form a T.
- Exhale and bend slowly to the right.

FIG. 2:

- Lower your right arm to your right shin and extend your left arm up toward the ceiling.
- Make sure your shoulders are in alignment, as though stacked over your right knee. Maintain an extension of the spine.
- Look up at your thumb if you can without straining. Breathe in and out slowly.
- As the left side of your body relaxes and opens up, slide your right hand further down your leg. To make sure your upper body stays in proper alignment, imagine you are sliding between two pieces of glass. Hold for several breaths.
- Feel your endurance grow. Envision yourself as a strong, stable, immobile triangle.
- To release, "pinwheel" your arms back up to a standing position.
- Rest and then reverse the pose.

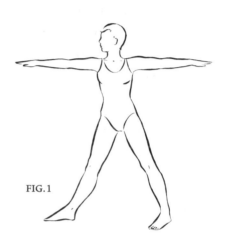

FIG. 1

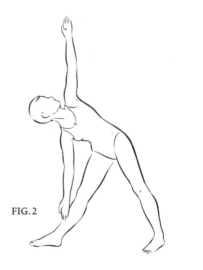

FIG. 2

MODIFIED PROUD WARRIOR
(Virabhadrasana I)

Modified Proud Warrior, a less intense pose than Proud Warrior (facing page), takes concentration and will-power. Doing this pose will improve your balance and increase your ability to concentrate. Use your steady breath as fuel to assist you in *Virabhadrasana I,* which looks a lot less intense than it actually is. This pose helps you realize that no matter what swirls around you, at your core you are balanced and strong.

- Stand with your feet directly below your hips, with your spine elongated. The shoulders are down and away from the ears.

- Step forward with your right foot, bending your right knee. Keep your knee directly over your ankle.

- Inhale and bring both arms forward, up, and overhead with palms facing each other.

- Engage your abdominal muscles 30 to 35 percent. Feel your breastbone lift away from your navel.

- Press your left heel into the floor. Keep your left leg absolutely straight.

- Gaze at a spot in front of you and breathe deeply. Hold for 8 to 10 seconds.

- To release the pose, step forward with your left foot.

- Repeat on the other side.

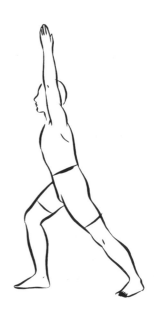

PROUD WARRIOR

(Virabhadrasana II)

An extension of Triangle, Proud Warrior (or "excellent" warrior in Sanskrit) is a slightly more advanced pose. It offers benefits similar to those offered by *Trikonasana,* or Triangle (page 63), with the added benefit of strengthening the leg and thigh muscles. Holding this pose reinforces the message throughout your body, mind, and spirit that you are a proud and fearless warrior, prepared to face whatever challenges may arise. As you become Proud Warrior, be aware that you can call on your inner strength and confidence throughout your day.

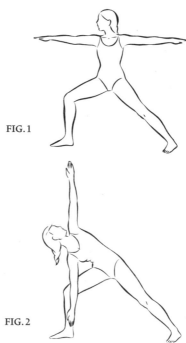

FIG. 1

FIG. 2

- Stand tall with your feet separated about 3 feet apart or the length of one leg.

- Turn your right foot out 90°; turn your left foot in toward the right about 30°.

- As you inhale, stretch your arms out from your shoulders so they form a T with the body.

FIG. 1:

- Bend your right knee, forming a right angle with your calf and thigh.

- Take care that your knee does not extend over the right foot. Your left leg is straight, with muscles engaged, and the sole of your left foot is grounded on the floor.

- Turn your head and gaze over your right hand. Shoulders are down and away from the ears.

FIG. 2:

- Bend at the waist as you "pinwheel" your upper torso to the right. If it feels more comfortable, place your right forearm on your right thighbone. Left arm is perpendicular to the floor. Turn your head to the left or gaze up at your raised left hand.

- As you grow stronger, lower your right hand onto a yoga block or as depicted in figure 2.

- Raise your left arm directly above the right. Hold for several breaths.

- Straighten your upper body and then your right leg. Lower your arms to your side.

- Turn your feet the opposite way and repeat on the left side.

ARCHER'S POSE

(Dhanurdhara Asana)

This pose strengthens the nerves and the leg muscles, opens the shoulder joints and chest, and increases concentration and focus. Not only will you look strong, but you will also become stronger—physically and mentally—as you assume the stance of a confident archer.

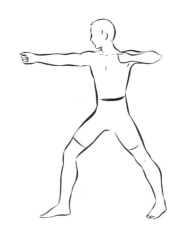

- Stand with your spine erect and your feet about 3 feet apart. Your shoulders are down and away from your ears.

- Turn your right foot out 90˚; turn your left foot in about 30˚.

- Keep your hips and shoulders facing forward. Bend your right knee so that it is directly over the ankle.

- Make fists and bring them to your upper chest. Straighten your right arm and look in that direction. Imagine there is a large bow in your right hand; with your left hand, pull back on the string. Make sure left shoulder does not round forward.

- Bend your right knee a little more and sink down, keeping your gaze fixed on the target. Keep your right knee positioned over the right ankle. With practice, you may be able to lower your hips so that your right thigh is parallel to the floor.

- Breathe slowly and deeply into the center of your chest. Engage your abdominal muscles 20 percent and pull back more with your left hand. Make sure your shoulders remain down and away from your ears. Hold for a minute.

- Lower your arms and straighten your legs.

- Reverse direction and repeat on the other side.

DANCER'S POSE
(*Natarajasana*)

This graceful pose strengthens and tones the leg muscles and tightens the muscles of the upper arms, hips, and buttocks. As is true for all the balance poses, it helps with concentration and focus as well as inner determination. Yes, you can be a lissome dancer . . . if only for those moments when you hold the pose.

- Stand erect with your spine elongated and your feet hip-width apart.

FIG. 1:

- Shift your weight onto your left foot.

- Inhale and raise your left arm with the palm facing forward, and hold your arm close by your left ear.

- Exhale and bend your right leg behind you. With your right hand, palm facing out, grasp the inside of your ankle. If it's more comfortable, you may grasp your leg with the palm facing in.

- The sole of your right foot faces up; your right knee points down.

FIG. 2:

- Inhale and focus on a spot on the floor in front of you. Exhale and very slowly lower your upper torso and left arm until nearly horizontal with the floor. Hinge at the waist.

- Raise your right leg behind you. Allow the right foot to press into your hand as you attempt to lift your toes toward the ceiling.

- Your body looks like a bow strung by an archer. Don't be concerned with the height of your raised leg—go for the stretch and balance. Breathe deeply and hold the pose for 10 seconds.

- On an inhalation, raise your upper torso and release your right leg and arms. Do the pose on the opposite side, then repeat on each side once more.

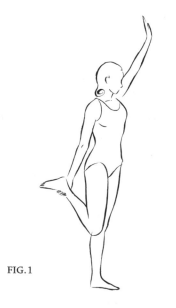

FIG. 1

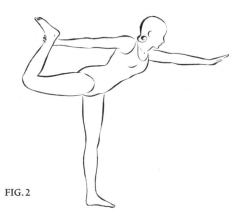

FIG. 2

STANDING HEAD-TO-KNEE
(Utthitta Hasta Padangusthasana)

This challenging pose will assist with balance and concentration. It stretches and strengthens the muscles of the legs, arms, and shoulders; works the abdomen; and stretches the back. Be patient but determined with this pose. Even if you only go as far as holding your hands beneath your knee, you will still experience a strengthening of the standing leg as well as improved balance. (See also Seated Head-to-Knee, page 105).

- Stand in Mountain pose (page 60).

- Shift your weight onto your left foot, establishing four-point contact between your toe and heel mounds and the floor.

- Engage the upper muscles of your left leg by pressing the thigh bone back toward the hamstring. Feel a lifting of the kneecap.

FIG. 1:

- Inhale and raise your right knee toward your chest; place both hands beneath your knee, interlacing your fingers. Make sure that you feel stable before continuing.

FIG. 2:

- Place both hands under the ball of your right foot. Maintain the lifting of the left kneecap. Gaze at a spot in front of you. Bring your right thigh toward your chest.

FIG. 3:

- Refocus your gaze and attempt to straighten your right leg until it is parallel to the floor.

- Bend at the elbows and pull back on the ball of your foot. With each exhalation, try to lower your upper body a little closer to your extended leg. Hold for a few breaths.

- Release by bending your knee and returning to an upright position. Release your hands.

- Repeat on the other side.

- Do one more round on each side.

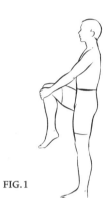

FIG. 1

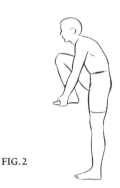

FIG. 2

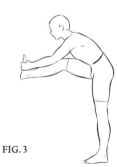

FIG. 3

STANDING SIDE STRETCH

(*Paravottanasana*)

This pose stretches and tones the hamstring muscles, back, shoulders, and arms. This is a strenuous posture, so be gentle with yourself. You may also discover that the pose is easier on one side than on the other. This pose presents an opportunity to accept yourself as you are.

- Stand with your spine elongated and your feet about 3 feet apart.

- Join your palms together behind your back in *Namasté*. If this is not possible, place your palms on opposite elbows or wrists.

- Rotate your right foot and entire upper body to the right so it is directed over your right leg. See that your knee is centered over the shinbone and not torqued to the left or right.

- Engage your right thigh to feel a lifting of the kneecap.

- Inhale. Lift out of your waist, creating a gentle backbend.

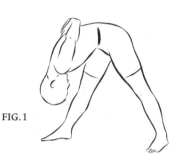

FIG. 1

FIG. 1:

- Exhale. Slowly bend forward from your hips, engaging your abdominal muscles. Fold over your right leg.

- Press evenly into the soles of your feet and feel yourself easing slowly into the part of the pose that feels perfect for you.

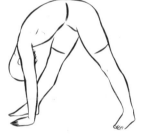

FIG. 2

- Allow your head to be heavy. Keep your chin tilted toward your chest and your hips parallel. Breathe deeply. With each exhalation, attempt to release further into the pose.

- Come up slowly, keeping your abdominal muscles engaged. Lift your chest 3 inches to flatten your back. Press evenly into both feet and continue to raise the upper body. Your head comes up last.

- Return to center.

- Repeat on the other side.

FIG. 2:

- If you need support, give yourself permission to bring your hands around to the front and onto the floor or your lower leg.

TREE

(Vrikshasana)

This noble pose reminds us of our connection to the earth, which sustains and nourishes all living beings. We spend so much of our time walking on floors and pavement that our link to the earth is weakened. The Tree improves your posture and helps stabilize the pelvis, elongate the spine, strengthen the legs and ankles, and increase flexibility of the inner thigh muscles. In addition, it helps with balance and centering.

- Stand erect with your eyes fixed on a focal point in front of you. If it is difficult to maintain your balance, you may also perform this pose while lying on your back.

FIG. 1:

- Bear the weight of your body on your right leg by tightening the thigh muscle.

- Inhale and raise your left leg, placing the sole of the foot onto the calf muscle or inner thigh of the standing leg. If your foot slips, hold your ankle with one hand.

- Stretch the inner groin of the bent leg by taking the knee out to the side, aligning the knee with the hip. Breathe deeply.

FIG. 2:

- Once you are balanced, you may raise your arms above your head or clasp your hands in *Namasté* at the center of the chest. If you are holding onto your leg, raise your other hand to the middle of the chest or rest your open palm at the heart center.

- Hold for 8 to 10 breaths.

- Return your raised leg to the floor and lower your arms.

- Repeat on the other side.

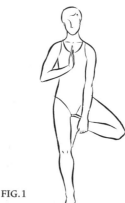

FIG. 1

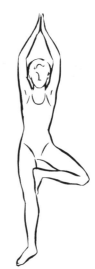

FIG. 2

BALANCING STICK

(*Tuladandasana*)

Balancing Stick will really get your system working. It tones and firms the legs, hips, buttocks, shoulders, and arms as it increases circulation and works the heart. It also improves concentration and balance. Focus on elongating the arms and leg when you are in this position.

- Stand with your feet together. Raise your arms over your head, palms together; if it feels comfortable, cross your thumbs.

FIG. 1:

- Inhale and step forward about a foot with your left leg. Point your right toe and rest it lightly on the floor behind you. Your heel is lifted.

FIG. 2:

- Gaze at a spot on the floor beyond you. Exhale and allow your upper body to pivot forward from your hip as your right leg lifts up straight behind you and your outstretched arms lower down in front of you. Your hips should be level. Viewed from the side, your body forms a T.

- If balance is a challenge, let your fingers rest lightly on a high-backed chair or shelf.

- Breathe normally and hold for 10 seconds.

- Lower your right leg and raise your arms, returning to start position. Check to make sure your shoulders are down away from the ears.

- Repeat on the other side.

- Do the pose once more on each side.

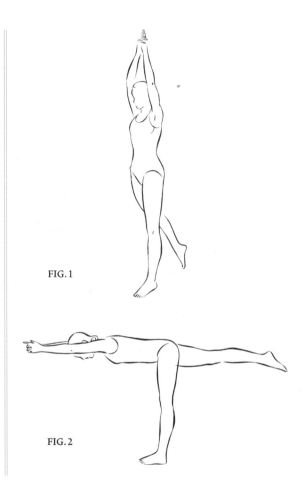

FIG. 1

FIG. 2

EAGLE
(Garudasana)

When you hold this pose, imagine that you are as strong and fearless as an eagle. This balancing pose greatly increases concentration. It also firms the upper arms, stretches the shoulders, opens the hips, and strengthens the thighs, calves, and knee and ankle joints. In addition, it works the abdominal muscles and brings a fresh supply of blood to the sexual organs and kidneys. (You may also wish to try Seated Eagle, page 93.)

FIG. 1:

- Stand with your feet together and your back straight and spine elongated.

- Stretch your arms out to both sides.

FIG. 2:

- Bring your left arm under the right, crossing both arms at the elbow. Place your hands together, palms facing each other.

- Pull your upper arms to your chest and bring your hands toward your face; if possible, allow your fingers to touch your nose and place your thumbs under your chin.

- Bend both knees slightly. To assist with balance, gaze at a spot in front of you and breathe deeply. Slowly cross your left leg over your right thigh. If you can, wrap your left foot around the right ankle or calf.

- Bend your right leg a little further. Your spine remains straight, and your hips are forward. Breathe deeply and hold for 10 to 15 seconds.

- If your balance falters, try to concentrate on your breathing and focus on the spot in front of you.

- Release your arms first and then uncross and straighten your legs.

- Repeat once more.

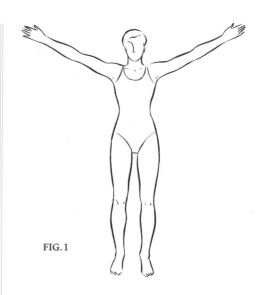

FIG. 1

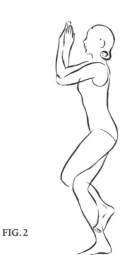

FIG. 2

CHAIR

(Utkatasana)

This energizing pose will make your body temperature and energy level soar. It will also work the thigh and calf muscles while strengthening the ankles and Achilles tendons. By rising onto the balls of your feet, you'll give your arches a welcome stretch too. Your legs will stay toned and strong while you improve your balance, focus, and concentration.

- Stand with your feet directly under your hips in Mountain (page 60). Arms and hands are held straight out in front at shoulder level. Keep your shoulders relaxed, back, and down.

FIG. 1:

- Inhale. On an exhalation, slowly begin lowering your body into a squat position as though you were about to sit in an imaginary chair. Do not go beyond 90° at the knees.

- Keep your feet flat on the floor, hip-width apart, with your knees over your ankles.

- Breathe slowly as you gaze beyond your arms. Keep your neck relaxed and extended.

- Raise your toes off the floor, rocking back on your heels. Hold for a count of 5 breaths.

- Return to a standing position with arms remaining at shoulder level.

FIG. 2:

- From this standing position, inhale and lift your heels off the floor.

- On an exhalation, slowly begin lowering your body into a squat position, again sitting in an imaginary chair. Do not go beyond 90° at the knees.

- Breathe deeply and hold for a count of 5.

- Inhale and raise back up to a standing position. Lower your arms and return to Mountain.

- Feel the energy course through your body.

- Repeat 3 more times.

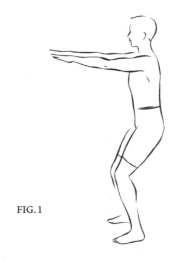

FIG. 1

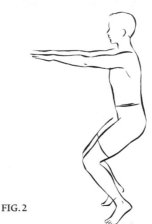

FIG. 2

VICTORY SQUAT

(Vijaya Asana)

Stand strong in Victory Squat and connect to your vital center of being—what the Japanese call *hara*—approximately 1 inch below the navel. Celebrate your power, determination, and focus. This pose strengthens the thigh muscles, upper arms, and abdominal muscles.

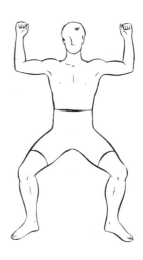

- Begin in Mountain pose (page 60), with arms by your sides.

- On an inhalation, step to the right so your feet are separated wider than your hips. Toes point out slightly. Exhale and bend your knees. Make sure your knees are over your ankles.

- Inhale and lift your arms up into a V position. Exhale as you lower and bend your elbows so your upper arms are parallel with the floor at shoulder level and your forearms are straight up, palms facing forward with fingers together. Your forearms and upper arms make a 45° angle.

- Your pelvis is neutral (not tipped forward or back), and your shoulders are down and away from the ears.

- Hold the pose for 4 to 6 breaths, feeling your "power center" grow stronger with each inhalation.

- Return to Mountain with your feet under your hips and arms by your sides.

- Repeat the squat. If you can, widen your stance and bend your knees a little more, taking care that your knees remain over the ankles.

- Repeat several times.

FORWARD BEND

(*Uttanasana*)

This refreshing pose stretches the entire spine, allowing the back to relax and the muscles to release. It loosens any stiffness held in the arms, shoulders, and neck and reduces fatigue and tension.

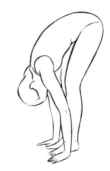

- Stand with your feet about 12 inches apart, with knees slightly bent. Arms are by your sides.
- Inhale. Exhale and bring your chin to your chest. As if you were an inflatable doll slowly losing its air, let your upper body sag. If necessary, bend the knees more so that your hands rest on either side of your feet on the floor.
- Let your upper body hang loosely like a rag doll.
- To come out of the pose, place your hands on your shins, knees, or thighs, depending on what is most comfortable for you. When returning to an upright position, lift the chin first. Don't come up with a straight back. On an inhalation, slowly uncurl up, one vertebra at a time. Elevate your body slowly to avoid any light-headedness.
- Once you're upright, gently relax your shoulders back and down.

FORWARD BEND WITH TWIST

(*Uttanasana*)

In addition to the benefits of Forward Bend, this pose gives the arms, shoulders, and muscles along the sides of the body an added stretch.

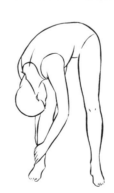

- Follow the directions for Forward Bend.
- Bring both hands to the outside of your right ankle. Feel a slight twist in the spine. Repeat to the left.
- Come out of the pose as in Forward Bend, taking care to slowly uncurl your spine so that the head comes up last.

SUPPORTED FORWARD BEND

(Upasthabdha Uttanasana)

This pose lengthens and aligns the spine, reduces lower back pain, and helps keep the back and neck flexible. It also stretches the backs of the legs and hamstring muscles. It is a relaxing pose that increases circulation and can relieve fatigue. You may find that using the wall for support allows you to let go and relax into the stretch for a deeper experience.

- Stand about a foot away from a wall. Your spine is elongated, and your feet are hip-distance apart.

FIG. 1:

- Allow your buttocks to lean against the wall. Bend forward, hinging at the hips. Bend your knees slightly.

- Reach around and use your hands to lift the flesh of your buttocks up and away from your sitting bones.

FIG. 2:

- Bend your arms and grasp your elbows with your hands. Allow your head to hang loosely between your bent arms.

- With each exhalation, see if your upper body relaxes a little bit more.

- Remain in the pose for 4 to 6 breaths.

- Straighten the arms. On an inhalation, slowly begin to come up one vertebra at a time. Elevate your chin from your chest to make sure the head comes up last and there is no strain on the neck or back.

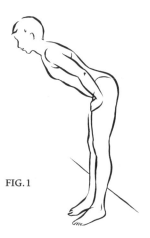

FIG. 1

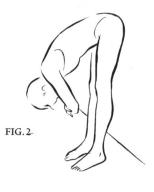

FIG. 2

YOGA MUDRA

(*Yoga Mudra*)

Mudra is a Sanskrit word meaning "seal." Yoga Mudra (pronounced *moo-dra*) is a symbolic gesture of yoga, in which the head surrenders to the heart. With your head held lower than your heart, you can let go and trust that it is the heart—rather than the mind—that truly understands. Yoga Mudra loosens the shoulders, arms, and spinal column, and improves posture and back problems. It also gives a great stretch to the backs of the thighs and brings a fresh supply of blood to the face and head.

FIG. 1:

- Stand with your feet parallel and hip-width apart. Clasp your hands behind you, interlacing the fingers. (If your shoulders are tight, hold a strap between your hands.)

FIG. 2:

- Bend your knees, tuck your chin toward your chest, and lower into a forward bend.

- With your hands still clasped, allow your arms to fall forward up over your lower or upper back without straining.

- Breathe slowly and rhythmically as you hold the pose for 6 counts.

- On an inhalation begin to raise your upper body, keeping your knees bent. Slowly raise your chin. Your head comes up last.

- When you have returned to an upright position, release your hands slowly, letting your arms float back to the sides of your body.

- Feel the release of tension in your neck, shoulders, and back.

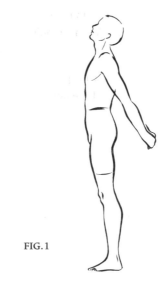

FIG. 1

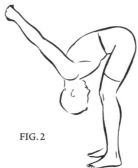

FIG. 2

SEPARATED LEG STRETCH

(Prasarvta Padottanasana)

This pose stretches the inner thighs, backs of legs, and back. It can help prevent sciatica, improve muscle tone, and increase flexibility in the legs and hips. It also massages the abdominal organs, aids digestion, and increases blood flow to the head and face.

- Stand tall with your spine elongated and feet parallel. Step to the right so your feet are wider than your hips, about 4 feet apart. The wider the feet, the easier the stretch. Your feet face forward and should not be turned out.

FIG. 1:

- Inhale and raise your arms to the sides at shoulder height, palms down. Shoulders are relaxed and down away from your ears. Bend your knees slightly to protect your lower back.

FIG. 2:

- Exhale and bend forward, hinging at the hips. Chin is tucked, and knees are soft. Slide your hands down the outside of your legs. Grasp your calves, ankles, or heels, if possible.

- Pull with your arms so that your head moves closer to the floor. Your elbows will bend. Feel the strengthening of your upper arms and shoulders.

- To make sure there is no strain on your neck, nod your head slightly as if saying, "Yes, yes."

- Straighten your back as much as possible. Lift your tailbone slightly, and if it feels comfortable, straighten your legs.

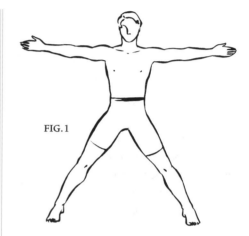

FIG. 1

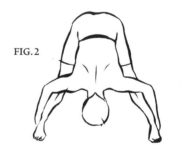

FIG. 2

- Remain in the pose for up to 10 seconds. Breathe.

- Prepare to return to a standing position by pressing your feet firmly into the floor and taking your arms out to the sides of your body. Keep your knees soft, raise your chin, and tighten your abdominal muscles. Come up with your arms out to the sides as if you were an airplane. Once your body is vertical, relax your arms by your sides in Mountain (page 60).

- Repeat the stretch once more. See if your head drops any further toward the floor the second time.

BENT KNEE PELVIC TILT

(Nikubjajanu Vastinirvlina)

This pose helps prevent and relieve lower back fatigue, strengthens the thigh and abdominal muscles, and helps promote an overall feeling of relaxation.

FIG. 1:

- Begin in Standing Pelvic Tilt (page 32).
- On an exhalation, tilt the pubic bone up and tailbone down by contracting your abdominal muscles. Inhale, pressing your lower back against the wall.

FIG. 2:

- To strengthen the muscles along the front of the thighs, bend your knees to your toleration point, attempting to bring your thighs parallel to the floor. The lower back continues to press against the wall. Hold for 10 to 20 seconds, breathing deeply.
- To release, slowly straighten your legs, engage the abdominal muscles, and press your hands into the wall to protect your lower back.

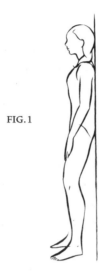

FIG. 1

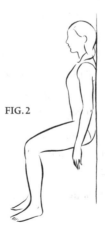

FIG. 2

ABDOMINAL LIFT
(Uddiyana Bandha)

In Sanskrit *uddiyana* means "flying up," and *bandha* means "lock." By tightly contracting, lifting, and holding the abdominal muscles, you create a lock in your body. Once you exhale completely, no air is being inhaled or exhaled. The movement of this posture tones the muscles of the abdomen as it stimulates the abdominal and intestinal organs. It also aids digestion and elimination. Always do this pose on an empty stomach.

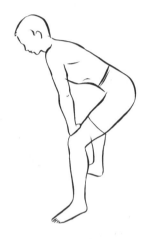

- Stand with your feet a little wider than hip-width apart. Your knees face outward and are slightly bent.

- Place your hands on your thighs with your fingers and thumbs facing in. Bend slightly at the waist.

- Inhale deeply. Exhale all the air completely out of the lungs.

- Lift the abdomen by pulling it in and up into the thoracic cavity, located at your solar plexus, between the navel and the breastbone.

- Keep the abdominal muscles contracted and while holding the breath out, "pump" the abdomen in and out forcefully and rhythmically. Remember that no air should come in or out of your nose or mouth. Continue until you need to take an inhalation.

- Repeat the cycle twice more.

BACKBEND

(Pratyak Uttana)

This gentle movement strengthens the lower back, increases flexibility of the spine, opens the chest, and expands lung capacity. Also it is an effective way of balancing the many forward-bending tasks we undertake during the day. If you are having a particularly stressful or strenuous day, Backbend will remove the psychological weight from your shoulders.

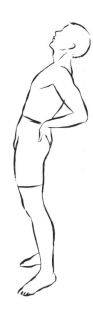

- Stand with your spine erect and elongated. Your shoulders are down and away from your ears. Legs are shoulder-width apart.

- Place the palms of your hands on your lower back with your fingers pointing down. Engage abdominal muscles.

- Inhale. Feel yourself lifting out of your waist and slowly lower your upper torso backward from the middle of your body. Don't allow your head to fall too far back, which can cause a strain on the neck. Keep your neck in line with your spine.

- Bend until you feel you are creating an extension of the spine, but without straining; do not bend backward too far. Keep abdominal muscles contracted. Keep chest lifted up.

- Hold for a slow count of 5, breathing normally. Your hands support the lower back.

- Slowly come out of the pose and return to an upright position.

- Repeat once or twice more.

Poses done from a kneeling position strengthen the thighs and stretch the spine. If kneeling on the floor or a mat is uncomfortable, fold a towel or blanket under your knees to provide some cushioning. As you do in the standing poses, align your body so that your spine is elongated; be aware of your legs, upper torso, back, shoulders, and neck. Let your breath be your guide as you hold the poses.

KNEELING YOGA MUDRA

(*Sidana Yoga Mudra*)

This kneeling version of Yoga Mudra (page 77) stretches and loosens the shoulders, arms, and back; improves the complexion; stimulates the nervous system; and relieves posture and back problems. Do not do this pose if you have high blood pressure or glaucoma.

FIG. 1:

- Sit in Thunderbolt (page 94) with knees slightly apart.

- Inhale and raise your arms in front of you, palms down.

- Exhale and bring your arms to the sides, with elbows high and chest open.

- Inhale and bring your hands behind your back, palms together. Interlace your fingers.

FIG. 2:

- Exhale and lift your tailbone, folding your torso over the thighs. If possible, allow your forehead to rest on the floor; your neck remains long and comfortable.

- Let your clasped hands fall as far from your back (toward the floor) as is comfortable.

- Only if your neck permits, lift your hips and come onto the crown of your head.

- Hold for 30 seconds to 1 minute.

- Lower your hips and arms, and return to an upright posture. Sit quietly, feeling the effects of this posture.

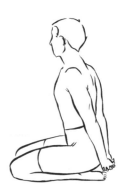

FIG. 1

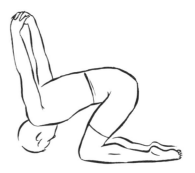

FIG. 2

BALANCING THE CAT I

(Bidala Tulana)

This essential pose helps improve balance, increases stamina, and aids concentration. It strengthens the arms, back, and legs and can help increase determination. Balancing the Cat will make you feel you can easily accomplish anything you put your mind to.

FIG. 1:

- Begin in "table position," with your knees under your hips and your arms under the shoulders.

FIG. 2:

- Focus on a spot on the mat, keeping your neck long. Inhale as you simultaneously lift your right leg straight behind you and lift your left arm straight in front of you. You are not aiming for height. What is important is that your leg is raised to hip level and your arm is level with the shoulder.

- Extend from the hip and shoulder. Internally rotate your right leg and foot (turn your toes to the left) to level the hips.

- Hold the pose for 30 to 60 seconds before returning to table position.

- Repeat on the opposite side.

- Do the pose once more on each side.

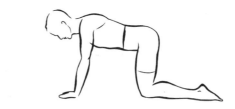

FIG. 1

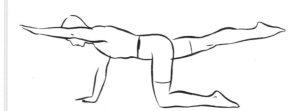

FIG. 2

BALANCING THE CAT II

(Dvitiya Bidala Tulana)

This pose will help improve your balance and increase your ability to focus. It firms and tones the buttocks and opens the chest. Follow this with Child pose (page 110), a good counterpose.

- Begin in "table position," with your arms under your shoulders and knees under your hips.

FIG. 1:

- Focus on a spot on your mat. Keep your neck long. Inhale; simultaneously lift your left leg straight behind you at hip level and your right arm straight in front of you at shoulder level. Internally rotate your left leg and foot (turning your toes to the right) to level the hips.

FIG. 2:

- Exhale and bend your left knee. Reach behind with your right hand and grasp your left foot. Use your hand to bring the foot back and up.

- Your heel should be *directly over* your left buttock, not pulled diagonally across your back.

- Tuck your chin slightly. Breathe.

- Continue to pull your foot back and up slightly as you hold the pose for 30 seconds to 1 minute.

- Lower your arm and leg back to table position.

- Reverse and repeat the pose on the opposite side.

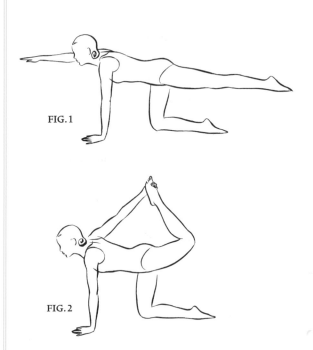

FIG. 1

FIG. 2

GATE
(*Parighasana*)

Gate pose stretches the muscles along the sides of the upper body and inner thighs as it tones the abdominal muscles, arms, and legs. It also stretches the muscles along the spine and back and relieves any strain in the neck and shoulders. This is an intense side stretch that needs to be done slowly and with concentration. Allow your steady exhalations to gradually deepen the stretch.

- Begin in a kneeling position with hands on hips.

FIG. 1:

- Exhale and extend your left foot out to the left side. Make sure your leg and foot are in line with the hip. Tighten the muscles along your left leg.

- Place your left hand on your extended leg. Slide it down toward your foot. Stop where you are most comfortable.

- On an inhalation, extend your right arm up and over your head. Your palm faces down. Extend out from your waist, feeling a stretch along the right side of the body.

FIG. 2:

- Look down toward your left foot.

- If you feel steady and strong enough, pull in your abdominal muscles slightly and look up toward your raised hand.

- Breathe deeply and with each exhalation, try to slide your hand a little further toward the foot.

- Hold for 4 to 6 breaths.

- On an inhalation, return to center.

- Repeat the pose on the opposite side.

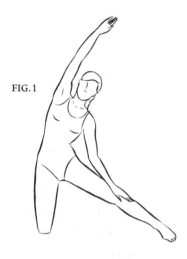

FIG. 1

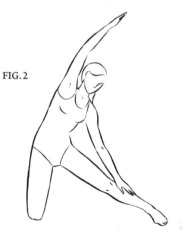

FIG. 2

KNEELING LUNGE
(*Anjaneyasana*)

This is the perfect pose to do if you spend a lot of time sitting. It lengthens the hip flexors and can relieve lower back pain. It also stretches the thigh muscles. Doing Kneeling Lunge relieves anxiety and tension while increasing energy and mental clarity.

- Kneel in "table position," with your arms under your shoulders and your knees under your hips.

FIG. 1:

- On an inhalation, move your right foot between both hands, then slide it slightly ahead of your hands.

- Exhale and bend your right knee to move both hips forward until your knee is fully bent without creating pain in the knee.

FIG. 2:

- Slide your foot forward so your shinbone is straight. Make sure your knee is directly over your ankle. Keep your palms flat on the floor; if this is not possible, make two fists and rest on your knuckles. Hang your head forward.

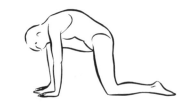

FIG. 1

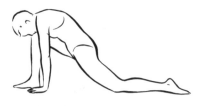

FIG. 2

- Breathe slowly; hold for 20 seconds to 1 minute. Feel the stretch across your left thigh through the hip crease into the lower back.

- Push on the floor with your hands to gently move back and out of the pose.

- Repeat on the left side.

KNEELING LUNGE WITH TWIST

(Saparivrttana Sidana Anjaneyasana)

This advanced modification offers the same benefits as Kneeling Lunge, with the added advantage of toning and trimming the waistline. It also helps improve balance.

- Follow the directions for the first 3 bullets of Kneeling Lunge (facing page).

FIG. 1:

- Inhale and raise your upper torso. Place both hands on your right knee.

- Exhale and deepen the lunge by lowering your hips without pinching (compressing) the lower back. Make sure your knee remains directly over your ankle.

- Place your left hand on the outside of your right knee and your right hand on the small of your back or over onto the left hip.

- Engage your abdominal muscles and turn your upper torso to the right. Gently gaze over your right shoulder.

- Return to center. Repeat on the opposite side.

FIG. 2:

- For a more challenging stretch, follow the directions described in the first 3 bullets above.

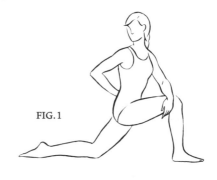

FIG. 1

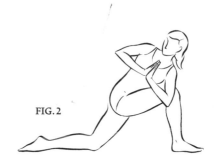

FIG. 2

- Bring your palms together in front of your breastbone in *Namasté*. Slowly rotate your upper body to the right and hook your left elbow outside the right knee.

- Exhale and gaze back at your right elbow.

- Breathe slowly and hold for 30 to 60 seconds.

- Return to center. Repeat on the opposite side.

CAMEL
(Ustrasana)

Camel pose gives an intense stretch to the front of the body and the spine. It relieves backache, helps correct rounded shoulders, strengthens the lower back, and stimulates the kidneys and thyroid gland. Do not practice this pose if you have high blood pressure, a herniated disk, or other lower back problems.

FIG. 1:

- Kneel with legs hip-width apart. Place your hands on either side of your lower back, fingers pointing down.

- Engage the abdominal muscles and move your hips forward as though they were pressing against an imaginary wall. Keep your neck in line with the spine and lift your chest upward.

- If you are a beginner, stay at this point until you feel comfortable with the pose.

FIG. 2:

- Curl your toes under to raise your heels. Engage your abdominal muscles.

- Inhale and lift the chest. Exhale and slowly bend the torso backward, sliding your hands down your buttocks and the backs of your legs and onto your raised heels.

- Continue to monitor your neck. You may want to keep your chin tucked slightly toward your chest.

- Inhale. Exhale as you continue to push the fronts of your thighs, hips, and abdomen forward.

- Breathe and hold the pose for 5 to 30 seconds.

- Come out by releasing one hand at a time.

- Rest in Child pose (page 110).

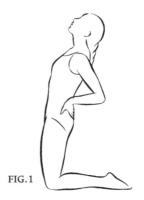

FIG. 1

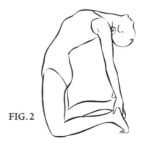

FIG. 2

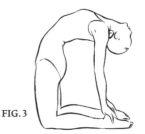

FIG. 3

FIG. 3:

- More advanced practitioners may wish to perform the pose with the tops of the feet resting on the floor, hands grasping the heels.

- Breathe and hold the pose 5 to 30 seconds.

- Rest in Child pose (page 110).

Seated Yoga Poses

Seated poses balance the energy of the standing poses. While they may be a little less strenuous than standing and kneeling postures, they are no less beneficial. Included in this section are a wide variety of seated poses designed to stretch, strengthen, and open different areas of the body.

Although most seated yoga positions are traditionally done on the floor, you may sit in a chair if it is more comfortable or if you're seated at your desk and want to incorporate some yoga into your workday. Many of the seated postures, breathing exercises, and meditations may be done from a seated position in a straight-backed armless chair. Here are a few guidelines for chair sitting:

- Sit in a chair with your spine elongated and your shoulders down and away from your ears. Attempt to use only the first 8 to 12 inches of the seat (so that you engage the back muscles).

- Place your feet on a cushion if they do not touch the floor so that your knees are level with your hips to help prevent slouching and strain on your lower back.

- Your chin should be level with the floor, slightly retracted so that you feel a lengthening in the back of your neck.

- Rest your hands on your knees, palms up or down.

If you wish to do these poses on the floor, sit on a mat or folded blanket for comfort. To ensure that your back is straight, you may wish to sit on a bolster or cushion. Whether you're in a chair or on the floor, always sit so that your spine is elongated, with shoulders back and down and chest open—and no slouching. Your hips face forward, as you perch on your sitting bones. Engage your abdominal muscles slightly to help keep your back straight. Imagine yourself seated on your throne of power.

EASY POSE
(*Sukhasana*)

Also known as Tailor Seat, this basic cross-legged seated posture is often used during meditation or breathing exercises. You may wish to sit on folded blankets or a cushion to bring your knees lower than your hips, to maintain the proper lower back curve, and to ensure that your spine remains straight and elongated.

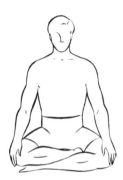

- Begin by sitting on the floor with your legs in front of you. Your spine is elongated. Your arms rest by your sides. Shoulders are down away from the ears.

- Cross your legs so that the arches of your feet are positioned beneath the outside of your calf muscles. Your right foot should be under the left knee, and your left foot should be under the right knee.

- Place your hands on your knees with your palms down. You may also place your hands palms up with the backs of your hands resting on your knees; lightly touch your thumbs and index fingers.

HALF LOTUS
(*Ardha Padmasana*)

Half Lotus is traditionally used during meditation and can be used when doing seated breathing exercises. Please note that we have not included the Full Lotus position because it can put too much strain on the knee joints. Advanced practitioners who wish to sit in Full Lotus should work with a yoga instructor to help prepare them for this strenuous position.

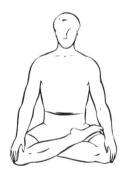

- Sit with your spine comfortably extended and your shoulders down and away from your ears.

- Place the sole of your right foot along the inside of your left thigh.

- Turn the top of your left foot so that it lies on the top of your right thigh. Be gentle with your knees and left ankle joint.

- Use a folded blanket or cushion to elevate your hips above the knees.

SQUATTING POSE
(*Nishadita Asana*)

This pose opens the pelvis and loosens the hips and lower back as it tones the abdominal muscles and aids elimination. Pressing the palms together firms and tones the chest muscles. It also stretches the Achilles tendons.

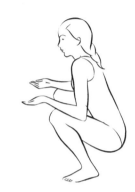

- Stand with your legs about hip-width apart.
- Bend your knees and squat. Hold onto the back of a chair if it is difficult to maintain your balance. For comfort, you may wish to separate your legs a bit more.
- Try to place the soles and heels of your feet flat on the floor. If that causes any discomfort, place a rolled towel under your heels or place a cushion under your buttocks.
- Pull in on your abdominal muscles.
- Rest your forearms on your knees with the palms open. If you prefer, put your palms together in *Namasté* in front of the heart center (breastbone) and press your palms together slightly.
- For an advanced stretch, place your elbows inside your knees and press against them, exerting a steady and smooth pressure.
- Hold the pose 1 to 2 minutes if comfortable, breathing deeply.

SEATED MOUNTAIN

(Upavishta Tadasana)

This pose strengthens the arms and elongates and aligns the spine. Because this variation of Mountain (page 60) is done from a seated position, you can easily make it a part of your workday.

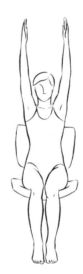

- Sit in any comfortable seated position either on the floor or in a chair. Your spine is elongated, and your shoulders are down and away from the ears.
- Inhale and raise your arms out to the side and up over your head, palms facing each other. Your hands may either be a few inches apart, or you can bring palms together.
- Stretch from the armpits. Inhale and exhale in slow, deep breaths.
- Hold for up to 10 breaths.
- On an exhalation, allow your arms to float back down to your sides.
- Repeat 1 to 2 more times.

SEATED HALF MOON

(Upavishta Ardha Chandrasana)

Make this variation of Half Moon (page 62) a part of your office routine. It stretches the muscles along the sides of the body and helps decrease tightness in the upper back and shoulders.

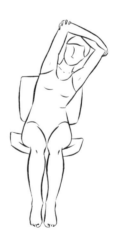

- Sit in a chair, with your spine elongated and your shoulders down and away from the ears.
- Inhale and raise your arms out to the sides and then up over your head. Bend your arms and grasp your elbows with your hands.
- Exhale, bend your upper body to the left. Feel a stretch along the right side of your body.
- Inhale and come back to center.
- Exhale and bend your body to the right, feeling the stretch along the left side of your body.
- Repeat 1 to 2 more times.

SEATED EAGLE

(Upavishta Garudasana)

A variation of Eagle (page 72), this is another seated pose that can be done any time of day. It stretches muscles along the upper arms and upper back, and releases any tension in the shoulders.

- Sit in any comfortable seated position on the floor or in a chair. Your spine is elongated, and your shoulders are down and away from your ears.

- Bring your left arm under your right, crossing both arms at the elbow. Place your hands together, palms facing each other. Your hands should be about 6 inches away from your face.

- Uncross your arms and give them a few gentle shakes.

- Bring your right arm under your left, crossing both arms at the elbow. Place your hands together, palms facing.

- When you're ready, release your arms and give them a few gentle shakes.

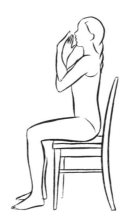

THUNDERBOLT

(Vajrasana)

Thunderbolt is used as a way to rest between poses—particularly the more strenuous ones. It improves the posture, promotes a deep sense of peace and serenity, and provides complete relaxation. Curling your toes under also stretches the toes and soles of the feet.

FIG. 1:

- Sit in a kneeling position with your buttocks on your heels and legs slightly apart. Face forward with your hands resting gently on your knees. You may wish to place a folded blanket or bolster across your calf muscles or at the backs of your knees. Take care not to impinge the knees.

- Attempt to have your big toes touching, heels angled outward.

- Close your eyes or gaze at a spot on the floor. Breathe deeply.

- Rest quietly in Thunderbolt.

FIG. 2:

- For an added stretch, raise your buttocks slightly off your heels and curl your toes under.

- Slowly sit back on your heels; the toes remain curled. Try to keep your spine straight.

- Breathe steadily and remain in the pose for up to 10 seconds, if possible; gradually increase to 30 seconds.

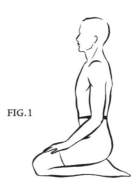

FIG. 1

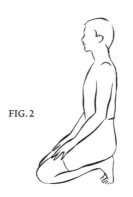

FIG. 2

HERO

(Virasana)

Hero pose opens the hips and hip joints and keeps the knees flexible. It massages the inner organs, helps reduce stiffness in the neck, and stretches the spine. It also is a deeply calming and relaxing posture. As you hold the pose, you may wish to reflect on a heroic figure in your life.

- Sit with your back straight, spine extended. If you are unable to sit comfortably while maintaining the curve in your lower back, sit on a folded blanket or towel (2 to 4 inches high). Have both sitting bones leaning into the floor or blanket.

FIG. 1:

- Cross your legs so that your right knee rests on top of your left knee.

- Place the palms of your hands on the soles of your feet.

- Move your feet away from your hips so that you feel a stretch in the hips.

FIG. 2:

- Inhale and make sure your spine is extended and that your shoulders are down and away from the ears.

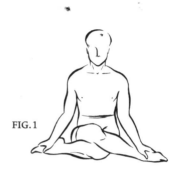

FIG. 1

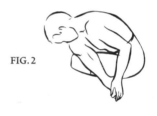

FIG. 2

- Exhale and fold your upper body down toward your knees; do not lift the sitting bones from the floor.

- Relax and breathe slowly.

- Return to an upright position and repeat with your left knee on your right knee.

HEAD OF COW

(Gomukhasana)

This pose (said to resemble a cow's head) is an effective way to counteract the forward-bending tasks that we do each day. Head of Cow stretches the spine, arms, shoulders, and neck and relieves tension in the upper back and shoulders. It also improves lung capacity.

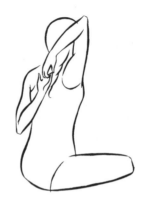

- Sit in any comfortable position on a mat or in a chair, or in Thunderbolt pose (page 94). Make sure your back is straight with your spine comfortably extended. Shoulders are relaxed and away from your ears. If you wish, you may also do this pose from a standing position, with your feet about hip-distance apart.

- With your left hand, reach behind your back from below; the palm is turned out, away from your body. Bend at the elbow, moving your hand up toward the center of your back as high as you can without straining.

- Raise your right arm beside your right ear. Bend at the elbow and reach over your right shoulder. Try to interlock the fingers of both hands or touch the fingertips.

- If it is difficult to interlock or touch your fingertips, grasp one end of a tie or scarf with your raised hand. Let the tie hang down your back and grasp the loose end with your other hand.

- Keep your body erect. Your right elbow should point straight up, not forward; your upper arm should be as close to your right ear as possible.

- Breathe normally. Hold the position for 8 to 10 seconds.

- Unlock hands (or release the lower end of the tie) and let your arms fall to the sides of your body. Shake out your hands and shrug your shoulders.

- Repeat on other side.

MODIFIED HEAD OF COW
(Vikrta Gomukhasana)

Head of Cow (facing page) is a strenuous pose, particularly for anyone who is not flexible in the shoulders. The modification below is equally beneficial but less arduous. It will give your shoulders and arms a great stretch. As an added benefit, it can be done anytime you feel tension or stress in your neck and shoulders.

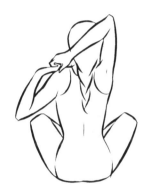

- Sit in any comfortable position on a mat or in a chair, or in Thunderbolt pose (page 94). Make sure your back is straight with your spine comfortably extended. Your shoulders are relaxed and away from your ears.

- Raise your right arm beside your right ear. Bend at the elbow and reach over your right shoulder. Your hand rests near the middle of your upper back.

- Raise your left arm to shoulder height, bending at the elbow; the palm faces out. Reach toward your right hand and interlock the fingers of both hands.

- Using gentle but steady pressure, allow your left hand to pull your right hand down and across, toward your left shoulder.

- Your left elbow points down to the floor as your right elbow points straight up. The upper right arm remains as close to your right ear as possible; your forearm is behind your head. Breathe and hold the stretch for 8 to 10 seconds.

- Release and reverse the stretch.

- Do the stretch a few more times on each side.

LION

(Simhasana)

It may not be pretty, but the Lion is a beneficial pose that helps tone and release tension around the facial muscles, jaw, and throat. It also brings a rich supply of blood to the throat and is said to help prevent colds and promote wellness. Do a few rounds of Lion whenever you are feeling tense, or when your energy level is low and your resistance is down.

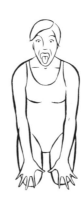

- Sit in any comfortable position on a mat or in a chair, or in Thunderbolt pose (page 94). Make sure your back is straight with your spine comfortably extended. Shoulders are relaxed and away from your ears.

- Place your open palms on your knees.

- Inhale. As you exhale, simultaneously open your eyes and mouth as wide as possible. Stick out your tongue as far as it will go.

- Stiffen your arms and fingers. Eyes look up toward your forehead.

- Exhale all the stale air from your lungs. Hold the breath out for 2 to 4 seconds.

- Inhale and slowly relax your tongue, facial muscles, arms, and hands.

- Relax and breathe normally.

- Repeat one more time.

TURTLE

(Kurmasana)

This pose stretches and increases flexibility in the upper thighs and groin muscles. Turtle also increases suppleness in the knees and hips and releases tension in the back, shoulders, and neck. Become like a turtle and go to a place deep inside yourself where you feel safe and protected.

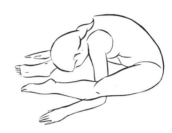

- Sit with your back straight, spine comfortably extended. Roll your shoulders down and away from your ears.

- Inhale and bend both legs. Separate your legs more than hip-distance apart. Exhale and allow your knees to lower toward the floor without straining, forcing, or bouncing. Allow the groin muscles to open gradually. For a more challenging stretch, bring the soles of your feet together, if it's comfortable.

- Thread your right arm along the floor under the right calf muscle, followed by the left arm under the left calf muscle. Palms are flat on the floor.

- Bend your upper body forward, rounding your back. Let your head hang heavy, with chin to chest. If it feels comfortable, allow your forearms to rest on the floor.

- Breathe deeply into the stretch. See if your groin muscles will let go a little more with each exhalation.

- Hold for 10 to 12 seconds.

- To release, inhale and bend your knees, bringing your arms out in front. Press your palms into the floor and walk your hands back toward your inner thighs to help lengthen your spine.

BOUND ANGLE

(Baddha Konasana)

Bound Angle provides an excellent stretch to the groin muscles, increases suppleness in the tendons and muscles of the knees and hips, and improves posture.

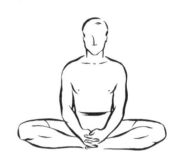

- Sit with your spine comfortably extended. Roll your shoulders down and away from your ears.

- Inhale and place the soles of your feet together; interlace your fingers around your toes.

- Exhale and lower your knees toward the floor without forcing the stretch. Use your exhalations to encourage your knees to drop just a little more.

- Breathe deeply into the stretch. See if you can allow the groin muscles to relax a little more with each exhalation. Don't bounce or strain.

- Hold the pose for 5 to 10 breaths.

SEATED ANGLE

(Upavishta Konasana)

This posture stretches the inner thigh muscles and the spine. *Upavishta Konasana* is beneficial for anyone involved in biking, running, dancing, and other activities that repeatedly work the hips and legs.

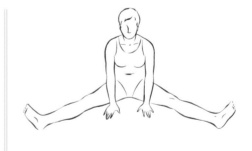

- Sit on a folded blanket or towel with your spine comfortably extended. Roll your shoulders down and away from your ears.

- Separate your legs a comfortable distance apart. Your toes and knees point to the ceiling and are not internally or externally rotated.

- Place your hands on the floor in front of you, with palms down. Elbows are soft.

- Inhale, keeping the spine extended. Exhale and bend forward, keeping the sitting bones on the floor. Your upper back remains flat and broad; your toes and knees point to the ceiling.

- With each exhalation, try to move your hands away from you a tiny bit further, bringing your upper body closer to the floor.

- Hold for 30 to 60 seconds.

KNEE ROCKING

This pose opens the groin muscles and improves flexibility in the hips. It also strengthens the arms, shoulders, and abdominals. Do it whenever you feel any tightness or discomfort in hips, pelvis, or upper thighs.

- Sit on a mat with both legs out in front of you and spine comfortably extended. Depending on how much flexibility you have in your hips, you may want to sit on a folded blanket or towel 2 to 4 inches in height.

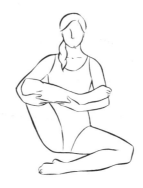

- Lift your right leg and bend it at the knee. Wrap your arms around the lower leg so that your right foot nestles in the crook of your left elbow or in your hand. Be gentle with your knee and don't force the movement. Cradle the leg with both arms and if you can, clasp your left and right hands.

- Use your arm to bring your leg toward your chest and abdomen.

- Keep your back straight and hold the leg as high and close to you as possible without straining.

- Moving from the hip joint, gently rock your leg back and forth in a sideways motion as though you were rocking a baby.

- After rocking your leg several times, switch leg positions and repeat with the left leg.

BENT KNEE SITTING FORWARD BEND

(Mahamudra)

This version of Sitting Forward Bend (facing page), with one knee bent, is a slightly less difficult pose and produces similar benefits. It stretches the hamstring muscles and the spinal column while massaging the abdominal organs. It also can relieve lower backache. Allow your body, mind, and spirit to perform this pose with a sense of acceptance and letting go.

- Sit with your spine erect.

FIG. 1:

- Extend your right leg. Bend your left leg at the knee and press the sole of your foot into the inner thigh of the extended right leg.

- On an inhalation raise your arms up over your head, with palms facing each other.

FIG. 2:

- Exhale; fold your upper body toward the thigh of your extended leg, hinging at the hips.

- Your back should be straight and not rounded, with the spine extended. Continue bending forward and stop when your upper back begins to round.

FIG. 3:

- Bend the extended right leg and hold onto the ball of the foot.

- Relax. Breathe into the stretch. Use your inhalations to help extend the spine by directing your breath to the upper chest. Feel yourself lift out of your waist.

- Exhale. On an inhalation, extend the spine and feel the lower back muscles stretch.

- Hold for 4 to 6 breaths. On an inhalation return to an upright position and release the bent leg.

- Repeat on the other side.

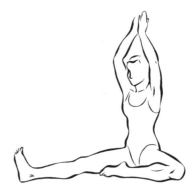

FIG. 1

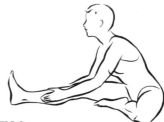

FIG. 2

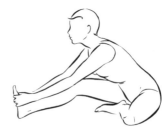

FIG. 3

SITTING FORWARD BEND

(*Paschimottanasana*)

This pose gives an intense stretch to your entire back and hamstring muscles as it increases flexibility in the spine and hips. By hinging at the hips and folding forward, your abdominal organs get a massage as well. Relax into the pose with a sense of serenity and surrender, allowing your flexibility to increase gradually.

• Sit with your spine extended.

FIG. 1:

• Lean forward, tipping your pelvis toward your thighs. If your back rounds, sit on a folded blanket or towel to maintain the proper curve in your lower back. Feet should be perpendicular to the legs.

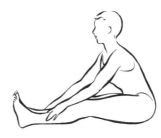

FIG. 1

• Bend your knees, and on an inhalation, reach down and hold onto your shin, ankle, or the balls of your feet.

• Exhale and begin to straighten your legs, bringing your upper body toward your thighs. Your back is straight and spine is lengthened. Knees remain slightly bent.

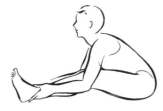

FIG. 2

• You may also loop a tie or scarf around the soles of your feet. Hold the ends of the scarf with your hands, keeping your knees slightly bent to feel the stretch in the lower back. Gently pull on your feet or scarf as you exhale and continue lowering your upper body toward your thighs.

FIG. 2:

• Relax, and with each exhalation allow your chest to sink toward your thighs without rounding your back. If you feel your back begin to round, stop. Look forward and out as you extend your upper body, keeping your neck in line with the spine.

• Breathe rhythmically. Do not strain.

• Hold for 5 to 10 breaths.

SEATED LEG STRETCH
(*Upavishtha Nalaka Uttana*)

This pose stretches the back of the legs, lengthens and strengthens the spine, and opens the hips. It increases circulation in the legs and is great for anyone with tight hamstring muscles. The difference between this pose and Bent Knee Sitting Forward Bend (page 102) is that you sit with the extended leg stretched out to the side rather than straight in front.

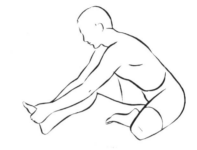

- Sit on the floor with your spine comfortably extended. If you are unable to maintain the proper curve in the lower back, sit on a folded blanket or towel, elevating the hips higher than the knees.

- Stretch your right leg out to the side; bend your left leg at the knee so the sole of your foot comes toward the opposite inner thigh.

- Turn your upper body to the right. Keep your spine straight. Gaze at your right foot.

- Bend your right knee slightly and grasp the sole of your right foot with both hands. If you can't do this comfortably, keep the knee bent and grasp your ankle or shin. Looping a tie or scarf around the foot can be helpful. Your upper back should be flat and broad.

- Hold for 3 to 5 breaths.

- Inhale and extend your spine out through the crown of your head. Do not stretch to the point of discomfort.

- Exhale and maintain the extension, keeping the upper back lifted and flat.

- Release the stretch. Relax.

- Switch legs and repeat the stretch on the other side.

SEATED HEAD-TO-KNEE

(*Janusirsasana*)

This stretch, a variation on Standing Head-to-Knee (page 68), increases flexibility in the spine and relieves discomfort in the back, shoulders, and neck. It can also help with sciatic pain. It massages the abdominal organs and restores a deep sense of calmness and a feeling of inner strength. Many of us have tight hip rotators and flexor muscles and may not be as flexible as we'd like. Don't force this stretch. Do a few rounds of Knee Rocking (page 101) before beginning to loosen the groin muscles and knee joints. Skip this pose if you are new to yoga.

- Sit with your back straight and spine comfortably extended. Relax your shoulders down and away from the ears. Both legs are extended on the floor in front of you.

FIG. 1:

- Inhale and bend your left leg. Place your left foot in the crook of your right elbow.

- Exhale and wrap your left arm around your left leg and interlace the fingers of both hands.

- Gently rock your leg side-to-side for 30 to 60 seconds.

FIG. 2:

- Inhale and press the heel of your right foot firmly into the floor. Exhale and, hinging at the hips, come forward. Bring your head toward your right knee.

- Inhale and lengthen along the spine. Exhale and pull gently on your bent leg, using it as a lever to bring the front of your body closer to your right thigh.

- Relax and deepen into the pose. Hold for 20 to 30 seconds.

- Come out of the pose and repeat on the opposite side.

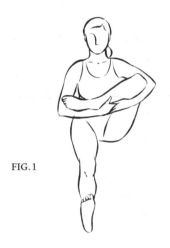

FIG. 1

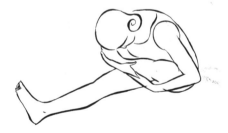

FIG. 2

SPINAL TWIST
(*Matsyendrasana*)

As you do this pose, try to get a sense of your spine rotating on its own axis. Spinal Twist stretches the spinal column and connecting nerves and helps reduce stiffness in the neck. It also massages the lower abdominal organs and aids elimination. When your body turns to the right, it is said you face the future; when you turn to the left, you review the past. Be open to what has yet to be and feel a sense of gratitude for what has come before.

• Sit with your spine extended. Legs are lengthened on the floor in front of you. If you are unable to sit comfortably maintaining the curve in your lower back, sit on a folded blanket or towel.

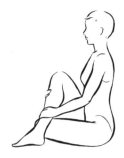

FIG. 1

FIG. 1:

• Bend your left leg; cross your right foot over your left thigh at midpoint.

FIG. 2:

• Inhale; bring your left arm around the outside of your right knee. Grasp your knee.

• Exhale; use your left arm for leverage by pressing against your leg and rotate your upper body to the right. Keep your shoulders level. Engage your abdominal muscles 15 to 20 percent to help protect your lower back.

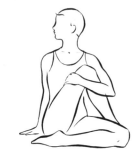

FIG. 2

• Place your right palm on the floor near your buttocks. Turn your head to the right and gaze over your right shoulder.

• With each inhalation, create an extension in your spine. On an exhalation, engage your abdominal muscles and slowly turn your body a little more to the right without straining the lower back. Hold for up to 1 minute.

• Release and return to center.

• Repeat on the left side.

MODIFIED SPINAL TWIST
(*Parivrtta Asana*)

This version of Spinal Twist (page 106) is a little easier to do because one leg remains extended on the floor. However, it provides the same benefits: it stretches the spinal column and connecting nerves and helps reduce stiffness in the neck.

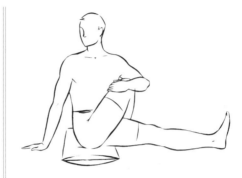

- Sit with your spine extended. Legs are straight on the floor in front of you. If your sitting bones lift off the floor, use folded blankets to elevate your hips.
- Bend your right knee and place the sole of your right foot to the outside of your left knee.
- Maintain an extension through the spine. Wrap your left arm around the bent right knee. Place your right hand on the floor by your hip or buttock.
- Use your right arm to help create an extension in the spine.
- Inhale and press into the right palm, extending out through the crown of the head.
- Exhale; engage the abdominal muscles and rotate your upper body slowly to the right.
- With each inhalation, create an extension in your spine. On an exhalation, engage your abdominal muscles and slowly turn your body a little more to the right without straining the lower back. Hold for up to 1 minute.
- Release and return to center.
- Repeat on the left side.

BOAT

(Navasana)

The more you perform Boat pose, the stronger you will become. This pose really works your "power center," the abdominal area, which is so important to maintaining a strong back. In addition to toning and strengthening the abdominal muscles, it strengthens your thighs and hip flexors and will greatly increase your stamina and determination.

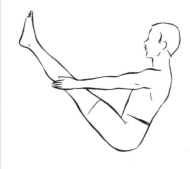

- Sit on the floor with your spine erect. Knees are bent, feet are flat on the floor.
- Bring your arms to the outside of your legs and grasp the backs of your thighs with your hands.
- Inhale and lean backward, balancing on your sitting bones. The tips of your toes remain on the floor.
- Your pelvis is in a neutral position (not tipped forward or backward). Exhale as you draw your navel in. Make sure the spine remains elongated.
- Inhale and lift your toes off the floor and straighten your legs. If this is too strenuous initially, keep your knees bent.
- When you feel balanced, release your hands from your thighs and straighten your arms alongside your legs, palms facing in.
- If your back begins to round, bend your legs slightly.
- Gaze toward your knees. Breathe.
- Hold for 8 to 10 seconds.

INCLINED PLANE

(Purvottanasana)

Inclined Plane stretches and lengthens the entire front of the body as it strengthens the wrists, arms, and shoulders. It firms the buttocks and thigh muscles. *Purvottanasana* also opens the neck, throat, and chest. Remember to breathe deeply to provide the necessary power, allowing you to maintain the pose.

FIG. 1:

- Sit on the floor with your legs extended. Your palms are flat on the floor behind you, fingers pointing away from your back.

FIG. 2:

- Lean back onto your palms. Inhale and raise your hips toward the ceiling. Contract the abdominal muscles and the buttocks.

- Exhale and slowly drop your head back. If you have any neck problems keep your chin tucked slightly toward the chest.

- Hold for several breaths.

- Bring your head up and gaze down at your feet. Hold for a few seconds.

- Lower your hips.

- Bring your arms to your sides and shake out your hands.

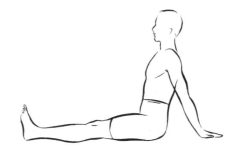

FIG. 1

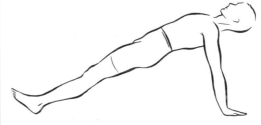

FIG. 2

Yoga poses done from a prone position (on your stomach) promote flexibility and strengthen the back and arms. Many also open the chest, stretch the abdominal muscles, and lengthen the hip flexors. The backbending positions massage and stimulate the kidneys. For obvious reasons, pregnant women should avoid prone positions.

Included in this section are several ancient poses such as Cobra, Bow, Full Locust, and Child (pages 111, 113, 116, 110 respectively), which have traditionally been part of hatha yoga for centuries. Because Bow and Full Locust can be strenuous poses even for seasoned practitioners, we've included the equally beneficial modifications, Cross Bow (page 112) and Half Locust (page 115) as well.

CHILD POSE
(Garbhasana)

This rejuvenating pose completely relaxes the back and neck and stretches the spine. Child pose massages the abdominal organs and promotes a sense of security and nurturing. It is a good counterpose to backbends.

- Kneel with your buttocks on or near your heels and with your legs slightly apart.

- Bend from the hips—forward and down—folding your upper body onto your thighs. The forehead rests on the floor or on a folded blanket or towel.

- Place your arms on the floor next to your legs, palms up. If you wish, you can also extend your arms on the floor in front of you, palms down, with elbows relaxed.

- Let your shoulders round.

- Breathe deeply and relax.

- Remain in the pose for 1 to 2 minutes.

- Raise your upper body and return to a kneeling position.

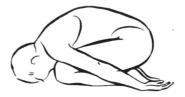

COBRA

(Bhujangasana)

As you go into this energizing pose, imagine a cobra as it rises and gets ready to strike. This pose tones the back, kidneys, and buttocks as it expands the rib cage, chest, and abdomen and firms the neck and throat. It also replenishes the lower back and pelvis with a fresh supply of blood and increases circulation.

FIG. 1:

- Lie facedown with your forehead on the mat. Your feet are comfortably close together with the toes pointing.
- Place your hands beneath your shoulders, palms down and elbows tucked next to the body.
- Engage your abdominal muscles and feel your hip creases press into the floor.

TO PREPARE FOR COBRA:

- Inhale; curl your upper body off the floor 2 to 3 inches as you *slowly* raise your forehead, nose, chin, shoulders, and chest. Your pelvis remains on the floor.

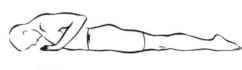

FIG. 1

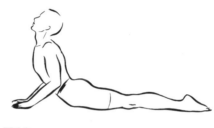

FIG. 2

- Lift your hands off the floor and feel your lower back muscles being strengthened. Hold for 3 breaths. Make sure your shoulders drop away from your ears.
- Place hands on the floor. Slowly release your upper body back onto the floor and rest. Turn your head to one side if you'd like.

FIG. 2:

- Return your hands beneath your shoulders, elbows bent and tucked next to the body.
- Engage your abdominal muscles and press both palms into the floor, slowly raising your forehead, nose, chin, shoulders, and chest off the floor. Shoulders are down and away from the ears. Keep your elbows bent at a 45° angle or less. Your navel remains on the floor.
- Lengthen your neck and gaze straight ahead. Hold for 3 to 5 breaths.
- Your upper body remains raised.
- If it feels comfortable, turn your head to the right and gaze back at your right heel. Hold for a moment. Lower your head and slowly turn it to the other side, gazing at your left heel.
- Return your head to the center. Exhale and slowly begin lowering your body from the waist, chest, chin, nose, and forehead.
- Pause and repeat.

CROSS BOW

The Cross Bow has benefits similar to those of the more arduous Bow, which follows, but it is a less intense pose. It massages the abdominal organs and improves digestion, stimulates the thyroid, opens the chest, strengthens the back and upper arms, and tones the thighs and buttocks.

- Lie on your stomach with your legs slightly apart. Turn your face to the right; the left cheek rests on the back of your left hand.

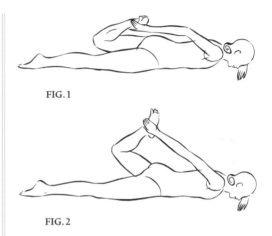

FIG. 1

FIG. 1:

- Bend your left knee, bringing your foot toward the buttocks. Reach back and across with your right hand, grasping your ankle or the front of your left foot. Be gentle to avoid impinging your knee.

- Your left heel goes in the direction of your right buttock. Lift your left knee an inch from the floor. Hold for a few breaths.

- Lower your left knee. Rest.

FIG. 2

FIG. 2:

- Raise your left knee and foot as high as you can, pressing your foot into your hand.

- Hold the pose, breathing deeply, for 20 to 30 seconds.

- Release. Reverse the pose.

- Repeat once more on each side.

- Relax in Child pose (page 110), a good counterpose.

BOW

(Dhanurasana)

Bow pose massages the abdominal organs and improves digestion, stimulates the thyroid, and opens the chest. It strengthens the back and arms and tones the thighs and buttocks. Attempt this pose only after you feel comfortable with Cobra (page 111), Half Locust (page 115), Full Locust (page 116), and Cross Bow (facing page). Do not do this pose if you have high blood pressure.

- Lie on your stomach with your chin resting on the floor and legs slightly apart.

FIG. 1:

- Bend both knees, bringing your heels toward the buttocks.

FIG. 2:

- Reach back with your hands and grasp your ankles (one at a time, if it's easier) or loop a strap around your ankles.

FIG. 3:

- Exhale and press your pubic bone down by engaging the abdominal muscles.

- Inhale and *slowly* raise your head, feet, knees, and thighs. Thighs remain parallel and knees are kept hip distance apart. Feel the shoulder blades squeezing together.

- *Gently* rock back and forth without pulling or straining. Breathe.

- Hold for 10 to 15 seconds.

- Exhale; release your hands. Slowly lower and straighten your legs.

- Relax in Child pose (page 110) or roll over onto your back and hug your knees to your chest (page 46); both are good counterposes.

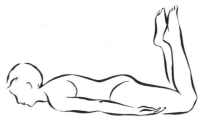

FIG. 1

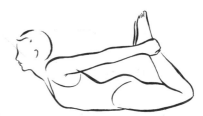

FIG. 2

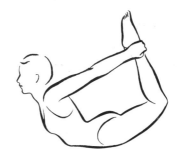

FIG. 3

UPWARD-FACING DOG

(Urdhva Mukhasana)

This posture keeps the back flexible and stimulates the nervous system. It strengthens the arms and wrists, can relieve back pain, and stretches the front of the body.

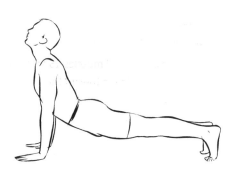

- Lie on your stomach with your legs extended straight behind you, with toes pointed.

- Bring your hands beside your shoulders, with palms down.

- Rest your forehead on the floor. You may curl your toes under or leave toes pointed, whichever is more comfortable.

- Inhale and push up with your arms to raise your head, shoulders, and chest off the ground. Engage and tighten your abdominal and thigh muscles.

- If possible, lift your knees off the floor without compromising your lower back, maintaining an extension. If you feel any discomfort in your lower back, place your hands on yoga blocks or on two telephone books. Throughout the pose, keep your breastbone lifted away from your navel.

- Roll your shoulders down away from your ears and raise your head upward. Allow your chest to open. Gaze up to the ceiling without compressing your neck.

- Keep lifting the front of your body. Breathe deeply.

- Hold for 3 to 5 breaths.

- Exhale and gradually roll down.

- Repeat once more.

HALF LOCUST

(Ardha Shalabhasana)

Half Locust tones and strengthens the lower back, buttocks, and backs of the thighs. It also helps relieve lower back and posture problems, stretches the hip flexors, energizes the nervous system, increases circulation, and improves concentration.

- Lie on your stomach with your chin resting on the floor. Legs are slightly apart. Your arms are alongside your body, palms down.

- Engage the abdominal muscles 15 to 20 percent. Extend your left big toe toward the wall behind you and then lift your left leg 2 inches off the floor. Keep the top of the left thighbone pressing into the floor so the left hip is not above the right hip. Focus on stretching and extending from the hip socket.

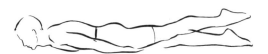

- With your leg still raised, breathe for a count of 5. Exhale and slowly lower the still-extended leg for a count of 5.

- Repeat with the same leg 3 times.

- Return your leg to the floor. Turn your head to one side and rest, breathing normally. Compare your left leg to your right and notice any differences.

- Repeat with your right leg.

FULL LOCUST

(Shalabhasana)

As does Half Locust, Full Locust tones and strengthens the lower back, buttocks, and backs of the thighs. This pose helps relieve lower back and posture problems, energizes the entire body, increases circulation, and improves concentration. It also firms the upper arms. A slightly more challenging pose than Half Locust, *Shalabhasana* improves inner determination and willpower.

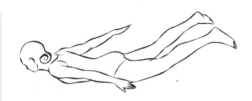

- Lie on your stomach with your chin resting on the floor. Legs are slightly apart.

- Bring your arms out to the sides in a T position.

- Point your toes and engage the muscles in your legs.

- Inhale deeply and simultaneously lift your legs, arms, shoulders, and head. Your head may come up in alignment with the arms; however, make sure the back of your neck does not feel pinched. (Instead of lifting your arms, you may wish to try making fists with both hands and placing them beneath your body at the inner groin. Inhale and lift both legs simultaneously. You may be able to lift a little higher, but remember, the emphasis is on lengthening.)

- Exhale and bring your arms back slightly, as if you were a jet plane.

- Remain in the posture for several breaths, imagining yourself soaring through the sky.

- Slowly lower your legs, arms, shoulders, and head.

- Relax, resting your head to the side for a few moments as you feel the energy stream through your body. Perform a few rounds of Windshield Wiper Legs (page 57).

- Repeat once more.

PIGEON

(Kapotasana)

This pose opens the hip area and chest; aligns the pelvis; and stretches the thighs, hip flexors, and hip rotators. It also increases circulation to the pelvic floor.

- Begin in "table position," with your arms under your shoulders and knees under your hips.

FIG. 1:

- Cross your left foot in front of the right knee. Slide and lengthen your right leg straight back. If the stretch is too intense, place a pillow under your left hip.

- Move the right side of your chest slightly to the left to align the hips, then lower your chest onto your left leg. Align your elbows under your shoulders.

- If the hip permits, place your elbows in front of your left knee or lower your body further. If you wish, extend your arms on the floor.

- Stay in your comfort zone as you feel a nice stretch in the left hip.

FIG. 2:

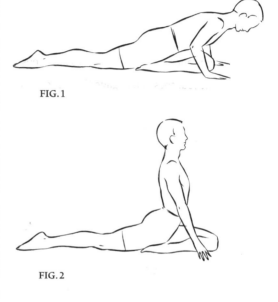

FIG. 1

FIG. 2

- Place both hands under your shoulders; press into the floor and lift the upper torso, raising your chest like a "puffy-chested pigeon." Keep your shoulders down and away from the ears. You should not experience any compression in your lower back.

- To release, come up onto your right knee or shinbone. Uncross your left leg, straighten it behind you, and shake the leg and foot a few times.

- Repeat on the opposite side.

FROG

(Manduka Asana)

Frog gives an intense stretch to the upper thigh muscles and helps increase range of motion in the hip joints. Do this posture carefully and with control. Take care not to overdo the stretch.

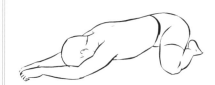

- Start in "table position," with your knees under your hips and your arms under the shoulders.

- Lower the arms so that your forearms rest on the floor. Make soft fists with your hands.

- Separate your knees a little wider than hip-width apart.

- Gently and slowly try to bring your buttocks back toward your feet. You may not go far; stretch only to your toleration point. Keep your lower back parallel to the floor. Engage the abdominal muscles to prevent a sway back.

- Move your hips forward so your upper body comes close to the floor. The weight of your body should be on your forearms Hold for a few moments.

- Slowly repeat this back and forth movement a few times. If the inner thighs permit, separate your knees a little wider to increase the stretch.

- When you feel ready, release by bringing your upper body forward and your knees closer together. Return to table position.

Supine poses are done while you're lying on your back. Begin by checking to see that your body is aligned. Briefly raise your head and look down the front of your body to ensure your hips are even and your legs are comfortably extended. Engage your abdominal muscles slightly and tilt your pelvis back to make sure the small of the back is on the floor. If your back still arches, either place a rolled-up towel or blanket under your knees or bend your legs, keeping the soles of your feet on the floor. If your chin and forehead are not level, place a folded towel under your neck to ensure that your chin does not poke up past your forehead.

Note: Pregnant women should limit the time they spend in supine positions after the fifth month (20 weeks) of pregnancy; or they should lie with a folded blanket or a pillow under the right hip, which displaces the weight of the uterus from the vena cava (a major vein that brings blood to the heart from the legs and pelvis).

THROUGH-THE-HOLE STRETCH
(*Avati Ayana*)

This stretch opens the hips and lubricates the hip joints as it massages and cleanses the inner abdominal organs. It also frees the shoulders and alleviates stiffness in the neck.

- Lie on your back with both knees bent. Your head remains on the floor.

FIG. 1:

- Cross your left leg so that the outside of the ankle rests on your right thigh. Bring your left arm through the space between your legs and around the right thigh. Clasp hands.

FIG. 2:

- Inhale. On the exhalation draw your right thigh toward your chest, lifting your right foot off the floor. Using your left elbow, move your left knee away from your body. Feel the stretch in the left hip rotator.

- Hold the stretch for several breaths. With each exhalation, see if you can draw your right thigh slightly closer to your body.

- Unclasp your hands; undo your legs.

- Repeat on the other side.

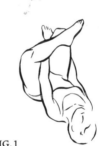

FIG. 1

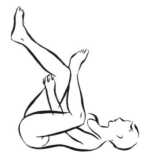

FIG. 2

BRIDGE
(*Setu Bandhasana*)

In Sanskrit, this pose translates as "forming a bridge." When you hold the pose, ask yourself how strong the bridge you are forming is. This pose increases flexibility in the back as it stretches and relieves tension in the neck and shoulders. It also strengthens the leg and gluteal muscles and opens the chest. You may wish to do Pelvic Lift (page 54) as a warm-up to Bridge pose.

FIG. 1:

- Lie on your back with your knees bent. Feet are parallel and hip-width apart; heels are near the buttocks. Arms are by your sides, with palms down.

- Inhale. Exhale and contract your abdominal muscles; curl your pelvis toward the ceiling, pressing both feet evenly into the floor. Breathe deeply.

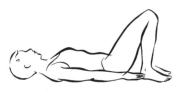

FIG. 1

FIG. 2:

- Inhale and slowly lift your lower, middle, and, if possible, upper back. Lift only as far as is comfortable. The weight is distributed between your shoulders and feet. The knees should be hip-distance apart. Feel both big toes leaning into the floor. Hold the pose and breathe deeply.

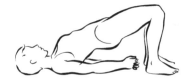

FIG. 2

- Walk your shoulder blades together and interlace your fingers beneath your raised buttocks. If that is not possible, grasp your ankles or use your hands to help prop up your hips and buttocks.

- With each exhalation, see if you can raise your pelvis a little higher. Hold until the pose feels complete.

- Exhale and release by lowering your spine back onto the floor *one vertebra at a time*. Relax.

SPIDER

(Supta Padangusthasana)

Spider pose gives an intense stretch to the back of the neck, hamstring muscles, and Achilles tendons. It can help relieve sciatic pain, and it massages the hips. It also helps with circulation and toning.

• Lie on your back with your legs extended.

FIG. 1:

• Bend your right knee and hug it to your chest for 10 to 15 seconds.

FIG. 2:

• Place your left hand firmly on your left thigh.

• Wrap the thumb and forefinger of your right hand around the big toe of your right foot. If this is not possible, use a strap or tie. Your left leg remains on the floor with the heel extended.

• Inhale. On the exhalation, slowly straighten your right leg vertically. If your hamstring muscle (on the back of the upper thigh) is tight, lower your leg to an angle less than 90°.

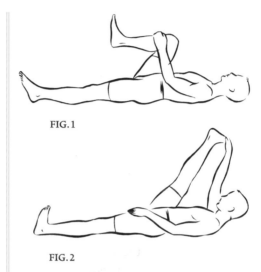

FIG. 1

FIG. 2

• If your neck permits, raise your forehead toward your knee. Keep a space between your chin and chest. Elongate the back of your neck.

• Hold the pose for 15 to 30 seconds. Slowly lower the leg.

• Repeat on the other side.

RECLINING SPINAL TWIST

(*Jathara Parivrittanasana*)

Reclining Spinal Twist is a centering pose that calms the mind and the nervous system as it balances the flow of energy throughout the body. It can relieve headaches and cleanse the digestive and elimination systems.

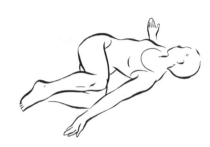

- Lie on your back.

- Bend both knees, with feet flat on the floor. Move your hips and buttocks 2 inches to the right and then bring your knees into your chest.

- Extend your arms out to the sides on the floor in a V position, palms up. Roll your legs and hips to the left, touching the floor. Your right foot is on the left foot; your right knee is on the left knee. Place a pillow between your knees if it is difficult to keep them together.

- If your back arches, move your knees closer to your ribs.

- Turn your palms up; angle your arms to 45° (in a V-shape) so your shoulders feel comfortable. Slowly turn your head to the right, away from your knees.

- Allow your back to relax. Hold for 30 to 60 seconds.

- Slowly roll your legs and head back to center. Repeat on the other side.

RECLINING SPINAL TWIST WITH EXTENDED LEGS

(Jathara Parivrittanasana)

This pose provides the same benefits as Reclining Spinal Twist but is a bit more challenging.

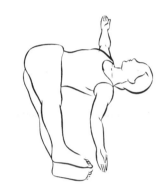

- Lie on your back with your knees bent and your feet flat on the floor. Move your hips to the right, approximately 2 inches.

- Your arms are in a T position by your sides, palms up.

- Inhale and draw your bent knees in toward your chest. Exhale and tighten your abdomen slightly; slowly lower your legs as a unit to the left onto the floor.

- Straighten both legs. Stack legs, one on top of the other.

- Turn your head to the right. Your head and both shoulders remain on the floor.

- Breathe deeply and hold the pose for 8 to 10 seconds, or until it feels complete to you.

- Bend your knees and on an inhalation, bring the knees back to your chest.

- Repeat on the other side.

RECLINING SPINAL TWIST WITH CROSSED LEGS

(*Jathara Parivrittanasana*)

If you would like a deeper twist, try this variation. Crossing your legs makes this a more challenging pose than Reclining Spinal Twist (page 122).

- Lie on your back with both knees bent. Cross your right leg over the left leg, slightly above the left knee.

- With your arms in a V position, palms up, slowly lower your legs to the left; your head turns to the right.

- Hold for 15 to 30 seconds.

- Return your legs to center and uncross them. Cross your left leg over the right and lower both legs to the right side; your head turns to the left.

- When you are ready, return to center and straighten both legs.

SUPPORTED FISH

(*Alambita Matsyasana*)

If Fish (facing page) does not feel comfortable, try Supported Fish instead. The benefits are the same and many people find it to be an even more relaxing pose than Fish. To be as comfortable as possible, use as many props as necessary.

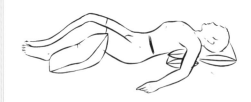

- Lie on your back, with legs extended and close together. Place a pillow under your knees.

- Place a bolster on the floor for your shoulder blades to rest on and a folded towel or blanket for your head.

- Lift your upper body onto your elbows and slowly lower your upper body so your shoulder blades rest on the bolster and the top of your head rests on the towel.

- Release your arms and bring your hands by your sides, a few feet from your body, palms facing up. Remain in this relaxing, expansive pose for as long as you wish.

FISH

(*Matsyasana*)

Fish pose is a great counterpose to Full or Half Shoulderstand (pages 131, 130). It opens the chest and compensates for forward-bending activities. It alleviates respiratory problems and stimulates the pancreas and pelvic organs. Pay attention to your neck throughout the pose. If you have any neck problems, consult a qualified yoga teacher before attempting this pose.

FIG. 1:

- Lie on your back, with your legs extended and close together.
- The hands are close together under your tailbone, palms down.

FIG. 2:

- On an inhalation, lift your upper body onto your elbows. Bend your neck backward, resting the crown of your head on the mat. Your back is arched; legs are passive. Make sure your weight is mainly on your elbows, not on your neck. Press both sitting bones firmly into the floor.
- Hold for several breaths.
- Return by pressing your elbows onto the floor. Gently lift your head, tuck your chin, and lower your upper body.

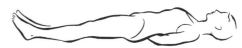

FIG. 1

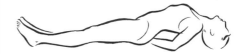

FIG. 2

CRAB
(Kulirana)

Crab strengthens the arms and wrists and firms and tones the hips, abdominal areas, and upper thighs. It opens the chest and throat and stimulates the solar plexus, between the navel and breastbone.

- Sit with your legs extended straight in front of you.

- Bend your knees with feet flat on the floor about hip-width apart. Place your hands slightly behind you, fingers turned out to either side.

- Inhale and lift your hips, making a table of your body from your knees to your shoulders.

- Exhale and let your head drop back gently as you release your jaw.

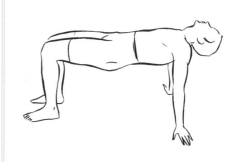

- Hold for 10 to 15 seconds. Breathe deeply, directing your breath to the solar plexus to increase your strength.

- To release, bring your head forward and tuck your chin. Lower your hips.

- Repeat once more.

CORPSE

(Shavasana)

Used between postures and at the end of a yoga session, this resting pose allows the body and mind to absorb the benefits of the previous poses. Since your body will cool down in this pose, you might want to wear socks and another layer of clothing.

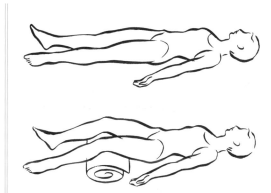

- Lie flat on your back. Your arms are by your sides, palms up.
- Keep your legs about a foot apart. If you feel any discomfort in the small of your back, place a bolster or rolled blanket under your knees.
- Close your eyes.
- Breathe deeply.
- Relax.
- Remain in Corpse pose for 3 to 5 minutes, or 5 minutes for every 30 minutes of practice.

Because we're usually in an upright position—whether walking, standing, or sitting—performing inverted postures refreshes, energizes, and stimulates the entire body. Inversions mitigate the effects of gravity, relieve pressure on the internal organs, and bring a fresh supply of oxygenated blood to the upper body, head, and brain. As a result, your complexion will glow and your concentration will improve. The increased blood flow helps remove toxins that build up in the organs and glands, greatly enhancing your body's flow of *prana*, or life force energy.

Modifications to some of the inverted poses are included. Keep in mind that they provide the same benefits as the more strenuous inversions, so there is no reason to push beyond your limits. Do not perform inverted poses if you have heart problems or high blood pressure. Women who are pregnant or menstruating should not perform some of these poses.

DOWNWARD DOG

(*Adho Mukhasana*)

This energizing pose aligns the spinal column, releases tension in the shoulders, and strengthens the arms and legs. It stretches and lengthens the hamstring muscles and Achilles tendons as well as increasing flexibility in the ankles. It also improves the complexion by bringing more blood into the face and head. Do not do this pose if you have glaucoma. If you wish, rest in Child pose (page 110) between the postures shown in figures 1 and 2.

FIG. 1:

- Begin in "table position," with your arms under your shoulders and your knees under your hips. (If your knees are too far back, you won't be in proper alignment when you straighten your legs and elbows.)

FIG. 2:

- Inhale; tuck your toes under. Exhale; straighten (but don't lock) your legs. Initially, keep your knees slightly bent to help extend the spine.

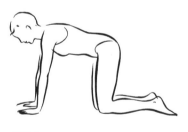

FIG. 1

- Push your palms down into the floor. Press your chest toward your thighs and shins. Visualize your tailbone extending toward the ceiling. Allow your ears to touch your upper arms so that your neck is free of tension.

- Breathe deeply as you hold the pose for 20 to 30 seconds. Heels may be off the floor.

- Keeping one knee bent, allow the heel of the other foot to proceed toward the floor; alternate one leg and then the other for several breaths.

FIG. 3:

- Raise your left leg straight up toward the ceiling. Don't allow the left hip to raise higher than the right hip. Rotate your left foot a few times in one direction and then the other. Alternate flexing your left foot and pointing your toes several times.

- Return your left leg to the floor.

- Raise your right leg, performing the same foot stretches.

- Lower your leg and return to table position.

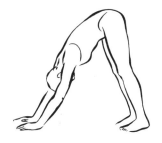

FIG. 2

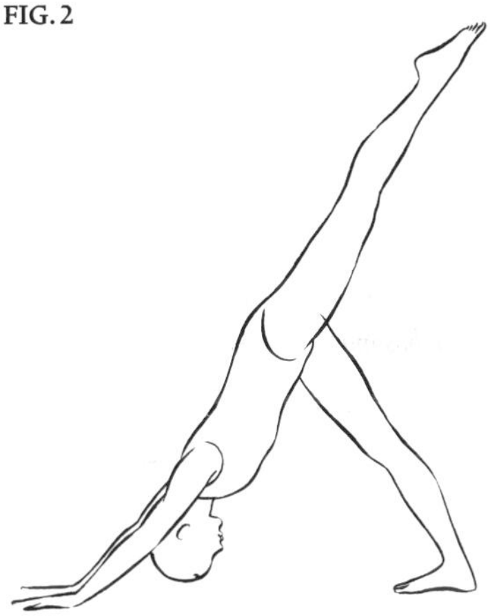

FIG. 3

HALF SHOULDERSTAND

(*Ardha Sarvangasana*)

Half Shoulderstand provides benefits similar to those of Full Shoulderstand (facing page) but requires less effort. It improves blood flow to the brain, nourishes the complexion, and stimulates the thyroid and parathyroid glands located in the neck, which control the metabolism. It also promotes calm and serenity. Warm up with Spinal Rocking (page 49) before performing the pose. Do not do this pose if you are menstruating or pregnant, have thyroid problems, high blood pressure, or glaucoma.

- Lie on your back with your legs extended on the floor, arms by your sides, palms down, head on the floor. Lift your head for a moment and look down your body to make sure it is in alignment.

FIG. 1:

- Bend your legs. Inhale and bring your knees toward your chest. Exhale and tighten your abdominal muscles. Inhale and roll your hips above your shoulders.

- Bend your elbows and use your hands to support your back at the hips. Let your hips rest into your hands. Do not put any weight on your neck or head. Make sure the weight of your body is placed on your upper back.

FIG. 2:

- Extend your legs over your head at a comfortable angle, not straight up. You should be able to see your toes. You may also bend your legs if that feels more comfortable. Initially, hold for 15 to 30 seconds. With consistent practice, work up to several minutes.

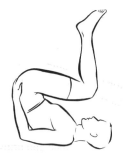

FIG. 1

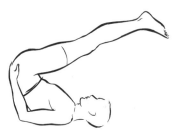

FIG. 2

- Release by bending your legs and slowly rolling back down. Use your abdominal muscles to help you come down safely. Be gentle with your lower back.

- Lie on your back and slowly turn your head from side to side a few times.

- Move into Fish pose (page 125) or Supported Fish (page 124) for a good counterpose.

FULL SHOULDERSTAND

(*Sarvangasana*)

Full Shoulderstand improves blood flow to the brain, nourishing the complexion. It stimulates the thyroid and parathyroid glands and promotes calm and serenity. If you have neck problems, consult a qualified yoga teacher before doing this pose. Do not perform this pose if you are menstruating or pregnant, have thyroid problems, high blood pressure, or glaucoma.

- Lie on your back, with your legs extended on the floor, arms by your sides and palms down. To prevent your neck from being compressed, fold firm blankets (2 to 3 inches thick) and place them under your neck, shoulders, and mid-back. Initially, place the top of your shoulders 3 inches from the edge of the blankets.

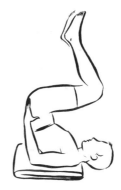

FIG. 1

FIG. 1:

- Bend your legs. Inhale. Exhale and bring your knees toward your chest. Your shoulders should now be positioned at the edge of the blankets, leaving sufficient room so that your neck is not compressed.

- Inhale again and roll your hips over the shoulders.

- "Walk" your shoulder blades toward one another.

- Bend the elbows. Use your hands to support your back at the waist.

FIG. 2:

- When you feel ready, extend your legs up vertically. Bring your hands higher on your back and move your elbows closer together.

- Stretch your legs and straighten your back. *Do not move your head.* Hold for 15 seconds to a few minutes, depending on your comfort level.

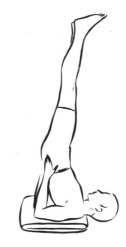

FIG. 2

- Release slowly by bending the legs and rolling the back down.

- Move into Fish pose (page 125) or Supported Fish (page 124) for a good counterpose.

PLOUGH

(Halasana)

Before attempting Plough, warm up with Spinal Rocking (page 49), Bridge (page 120), and Half or Full Shoulderstand (pages 130, 131). Beginners should rest their toes on the seat of a chair rather than on the floor. Like other inverted poses, the Plough improves blood flow to the brain and nourishes the complexion. It stimulates the thyroid and parathyroid glands in the neck and promotes calm and serenity. It also stretches the muscles along the back of the legs. Do not do this pose if you are menstruating or pregnant or if you have thyroid problems, high blood pressure, glaucoma, or disc injuries.

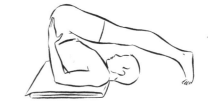

- To prevent compression of the neck, use blankets as described in Full Shoulderstand (page 131). Lie on your back with your shoulders positioned 3 inches from the edge of the blankets. Your legs extended on the floor, arms beside your body, palms down. Your head is on the floor. Lift your head for a moment to make sure your body is aligned.

- Bend your legs. Inhale. Exhale and bring your knees toward your chest.

- Inhale and slowly raise both legs over your head, pushing your palms against the floor. Bend your elbows, bringing your hands onto your lower back to support your hips. Your shoulders should now be at the edge of the blankets with no restriction in your neck.

- Exhale and slowly lower your legs behind your head in the direction of the floor; it is important to keep your back straight and move with control. Initially, rest your toes on a chair, pillow, or folded blanket. Once you feel comfortable, you can rest the tops of your toes lightly on the floor. Keep your legs straight. If you feel any discomfort in your neck, head, or lower back, come out of the pose and check that your body is aligned and properly supported on blankets.

- Remain in this position for 15 to 30 seconds at first, eventually working up to 1 to 2 minutes.

- To come out of the pose, bend your knees and bring them to your forehead.

- Gently and slowly roll down, taking care that there is no strain on your lower back. Allow your hands to continue to support your back the entire way down to the floor.

- Relax in Corpse pose (page 127).

LEGS-AGAINST-WALL

(*Viparita Karani*)

This simple inversion—as well as the modification that follows—relieves swollen and tired feet and improves circulation in the legs and hips. It also has a calming effect on the nervous system and may relieve menstrual difficulties and PMS. This is a good pose if you want to do inversions when menstruating. Breathe deeply and enjoy its restorative effects.

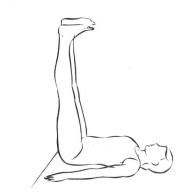

- Lie on your right side with knees bent and thighs near your chest. Position the upper body perpendicular to the wall with the buttocks and soles of the feet touching the wall.

- Inhale and swing both legs up so they rest on the wall. Exhale.

- Buttocks should be as close to the wall as possible. Arms are on the floor in a V position or stretched out from the shoulders in a T position, palms up.

- You should not feel any discomfort in the lower back. Make any adjustments to your position to feel comfortable.

- Stay in the pose for 5 to 10 minutes. If you feel "pins and needles" in your feet, bend and straighten your legs a few times. If uncomfortable sensations persist, come out of the posture.

LEGS-ON-CHAIR

(*Asanasthita Jangha*)

This modification provides the same benefits as Legs-Against-Wall. It may be easier, however, for some people to get their legs onto a chair rather than against a wall. This relaxing pose also provides some variety to your yoga routine. Before you begin, place a chair at the end of your mat or blanket.

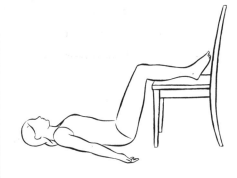

- Lie on your back with your arms comfortably by your sides, with palms up.

- Slide your body close to the chair. Lift your feet from the floor and place them on the chair so that your heels and backs of calves rest on the seat.

- Remain in this comfortable pose for as long as you wish, breathing deeply.

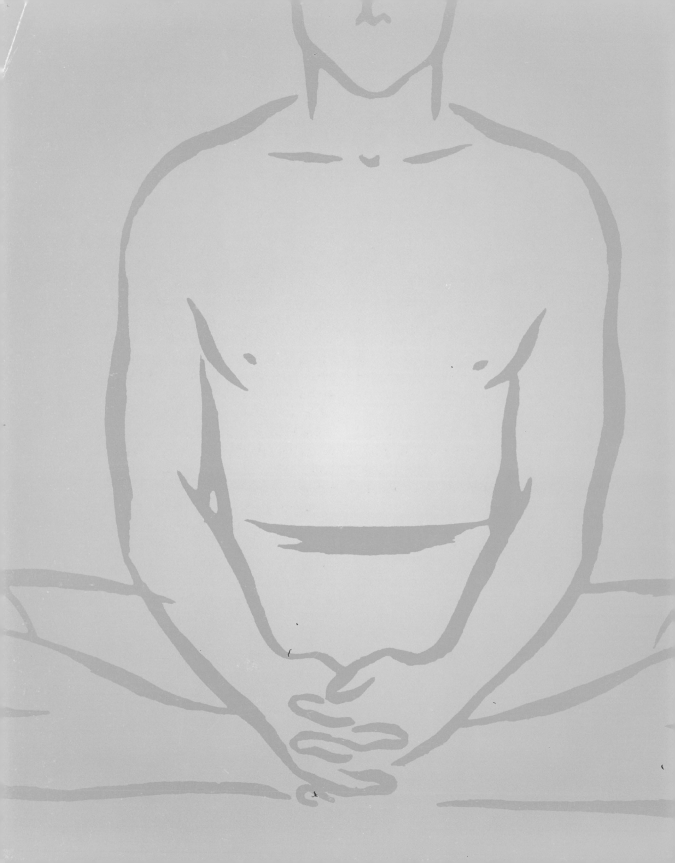

4

MEDITATIONS

A MIND TOO ACTIVE IS NO MIND AT ALL.
—*Theodore Roethke*

Although there is no rule that says you should do yoga and meditation together, many people find that meditation completes and complements their yoga practice. Think of it as a three-part harmony: yoga postures (*asanas*), deep breathing (*pranayama*), and meditation (*dhyana*), all designed to bring you into the present moment.

The positive effects of meditation are well documented: heart and respiration rate slow, blood pressure drops, and the physical symptoms of stress decrease as your body relaxes. Meditation helps still the mind, calm the emotions, and promote peace and serenity. Although we may be aware of these benefits, for many of us it is a challenge to sit and be still. "I can't find the time." "I've tried meditation but couldn't concentrate, so I gave up." "I just can't sit still for that long." Sound familiar? We hope that the 10 meditations that follow will help introduce, reintroduce, or reinforce a regular meditation practice.

It has been said that to meditate, we need three things: great faith, great perseverance, and great questions. Some practical considerations are involved as well. Before meditating, it helps to get ready,

physically and emotionally. Sitting to meditate without preparing your body and mind first is like stopping a car with the engine still racing. Hatha yoga began as a way for yogis to prepare themselves for the physical demands of meditation. Enhance your meditation practice by emulating the masters: perform some yoga postures and deep breathing exercises to help relax your body and mind and bring you into the present (rather than rehashing what already happened yesterday or preparing for what might happen tomorrow).

Find a quiet place where you won't be disturbed. Some people enjoy soft music or the sound of chimes or a table fountain; others prefer silence. Try it various ways and see what works best for you. Unless noted otherwise, sit in an upright position for meditation. If you are seated on a blanket or a mat on the floor, using a cushion will help keep your spine extended. Sit in Easy pose (page 90), Thunderbolt (page 94), or any other sitting posture that is comfortable for you. If you would rather be seated in a chair, take care that your spine is comfortably elongated and your knees are level with your hips (see introduction to seated poses, page 89). Make sure your shoulders are relaxed and down away from your ears. Your eyes may be closed or cast downward.

Rest the backs of your hands on your knees or in your lap, with fingers slightly curled. You may wish to hold your hands in what is known as a hand mudra (below). *Jnana mudra*, or "knowledge gesture," is often used to enhance concentration. This classic hand gesture, which represents the union of human and divine consciousness, is made by gently touching tips of the thumbs and index fingers, completing an energy circuit in the body.

Should you need to lie down during meditation choose either Legs-Against-Wall (page 133) or Corpse (page 127). In Corpse pose, place a rolled towel or bolster beneath the backs of your knees so there is no strain or discomfort in your back. If you fall asleep, don't worry: you probably need the rest. If you continue to fall asleep, however, you may wish to try seated meditation.

We have also included a walking meditation, a more active meditation that is performed slowly, deliberately, and with focus. This may be easier for you in general, or you may wish to try it occasionally as an alternative to sitting still. Because chanting is an effective way to release energy and help with concentration, a meditation that focuses on the sound of *Om* is included on page 141.

When meditating, it may be helpful to focus externally: on an object, sound, counting, mantra, image, or icon. You might try to focus internally, simply following your breath and repeating silently, "Breathing in, breathing out." You may wish to focus on a word such as *peace, amen,* or *shalom.* When thoughts arise—and they will—return to your breathing. If you feel uncomfortable, shift positions, moving slowly and with awareness. Don't just "tough it out." You want your practice to be pleasant and peaceful, not punishing.

If you are new to meditation, try it for 10 minutes at first; gradually, increase the time in 5-minute increments. With practice, determination, and patience, you will eventually be able to expand the time spent in meditation and ultimately experience the profound physical, emotional, mental, and spiritual benefits that can result from sitting in quiet contemplation.

Please note that the 10 meditations that follow are meant as recommendations. Some may work for you, while others may not. Continue using your favorite meditation if you have one, or use these as an inspiration to create some new meditations.

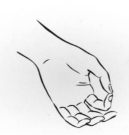

CANDLE GAZING MEDITATION

Many people find that gazing at a candle helps them to concentrate. Create your own sacred ritual through candle gazing.

- Light a candle and sit before it, either cross-legged on a cushion or in a chair with your feet flat on the floor and your spine comfortably extended.

- Breathe in and out.

- Gaze at the candle's flame as you allow your breath to deepen and slow. Focus on the flame. Do not blink.

- When you feel ready, close your eyes. Focus on the image of the flame that you see on the inside of your eyelids.

- Continue to breathe deeply, focusing on the image.

- As the image begins to change and recede, imagine your essence merging with the candle's energy, lighting a pathway to a place of complete happiness and serenity.

- When the candle image evaporates and finally disappears, invite your joyful spirit into this expansive place of happiness.

MEDITATION OF CONNECTION

"When, before the beauty of a sunset or a mountain, you pause and exclaim, 'Ah,' you are participating in divinity," wrote Joseph Campbell. We have all experienced those moments of intense connection to something greater than ourselves. However we define it, when that connection occurs we are transported to a place of profound wonder, peace, and beauty.

- Picture an awe-inspiring natural place. It may be an actual place that you have visited or seen in a picture or a place that exists only in your mind's eye.

- Go to that place and look around. Do you see plants or flowers? Are animal companions nearby? Do you hear any sounds? Is the sun rising or setting?

- Breathe deeply as you connect to your special place.

- Inhale and repeat silently: *I stand in awe of the beauty and grace.*

- Exhale and repeat silently: *That is the natural world.*

- Inhale and say: *Beauty and grace.*

- Exhale and say: *Natural world.*

- Dwell in your peaceful sanctuary for as long as you like, repeating these simple thoughts.

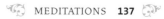

LOTUS FLOWER MEDITATION

The lotus flower has long been a symbol of perfection, purity, and simplicity. The thousand-petal lotus is often associated with cosmic consciousness, divine light, or the higher mind. While the lotus blossom represents perfection and purity, its roots remain firmly grounded in the dirt. Without the basic element of earth, the plant could not survive, grow, or blossom. The lotus flower reminds us that while we may strive for higher awareness from above, we can't forget our vital connection to the physical earth below.

- Sit in any comfortable position with your spine extended. Close your eyes.
- Breathe deeply as you envision a glorious thousand-petal lotus blossom.
- Inhale and imagine the lotus blossom growing in your heart center. This center is the bridge between the 3 lower physical centers of energy, or *chakras*, and the 3 higher spiritual *chakras*.
- Exhale and acknowledge the connection between your physical body and cosmic consciousness.
- Breathe deeply and with each exhalation allow the lotus flower to keep unfolding.
- Go deep within and gaze at the beautiful open flower. Note that a gift—an image, an insight, a message, or a vision—awaits you.
- Ask yourself: *What gift does the lotus flower hold for me?*
- Continue breathing, focusing on the precious gift that the Lotus Flower of Your Heart has brought you. What use will you make of this gift?
- Place the gift in a secret, safe place within. Know that it remains there for you whenever you need it.

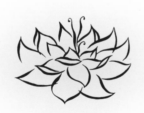

MINDFULNESS MEDITATION

This meditation uses external sound to help maintain focus and concentration. In the book *Peace Is Every Step*, author Thich Nhat Hanh explains that in his Buddhist tradition, temple bells are used as reminders to stop, reflect, and breathe. Sometimes a verse is recited: "Listen, listen. This wonderful sound brings me back to my true self." Allow the sound of a ringing bell or chime to be a reminder to pause, become aware of your breath, and return to that quiet place within. Do this anywhere and anytime you hear a bell.

- Sit in any comfortable position with your spine comfortably extended.
- In front of you, place a small bell or chime that makes a pleasant ringing sound when struck.
- Lower or close your eyes.
- Ring the bell or strike the chime.
- Inhale and focus on the clear sound of the bell. Allow other sounds to fall away.
- Exhale and listen as the sound begins to fade and then stops.
- Breathe in and out. Listen to the silence that exists where sound was before.
- Ring the bell once again. See if you can inhale for the duration of the ringing.
- When the sound stops, hold your breath for a moment and attend to the silence of the nonringing.
- Exhale deeply. When complete, hold your breath out for a moment.
- Allow your breath to return to normal as you focus on the thought:
  In silence I become aware of my true self.

NAMAHA MEDITATION

Many of us are familiar with *Namasté*, the Sanskrit word indicating respect, which means "I bow to the divine in you" or "I greet the light in you." *Namaha*, a lesser-known Sanskrit word, means "Not me" or "It is not about me." It reflects the notion that we are not the ones in control. During those inevitable times when we feel lost or confused and don't know which way to turn, or when our best-made plans go awry, trust that all is as it should be and remember, *Namaha*.

- Inhale and repeat silently: *It is not about me. Namaha.*

- Exhale and repeat silently: *All is well. Namaha.*

- Inhale and repeat silently: *There is a greater plan. Namaha.*

- Exhale and repeat silently: *I have faith. Namaha.*

- As you continue to inhale and exhale, simply repeat *Namaha* until its meaning fades and its essence fills your consciousness.

OCEAN MEDITATION

For many of us, nothing is more restorative, calming, and peaceful than gazing at the waves and listening to the sound of the ocean. It is the place we go to feel rejuvenated, inspired, and alive. Become aware of the endless cycle of the tides as you allow the ocean to soothe your body, mind, and spirit.

- On an inhalation, visualize a calm ocean scene.

- Exhale. Hear the gentle waves. Use Sounding Breath (page 28) as you exhale to mimic the sound of the calm waters.

- Focus on this ocean scene as you continue inhaling and exhaling to the rhythm of the tide. Feel the breeze. Smell the salt-laden air. Hear the cries of the gulls overhead. Melt as the sun's warmth caresses your skin.

- Inhale and breathe in the restorative energy of the ocean. Allow its healing and calming properties to wash through you and over you.

- Exhale, expelling tension and stress. Watch them float out to sea and disappear over the horizon.

- Breathe in health and well-being.

- Breathe out anxiety and worry.

- Continue breathing in this manner until you feel completely drained of tension and filled with peace. Imagine you are as placid as the ocean at slack tide.

OM MEDITATION

Om (ॐ) is the sound of all sounds, the sacred sound of the Universe, the sound of creation. It has been said that the sound of *Om* is the closest the human voice can get to the sound of the universal vibration. If you feel self-conscious, start by repeating "*Om*" silently at first. As you feel more comfortable, begin chanting aloud, gradually increasing the volume. Repeating the sound of *Om* is a great way to release tension. Feel the vibration move from your abdominal area, into your chest and throat, up to your forehead, and out the crown of your head as the sound connects to universal consciousness. Remember that the sound of *Om* is composed of 4 parts: *ah* (corresponding to the waking state); *oh* (corresponding to the dreaming state); *mmm* (corresponding to the deep sleeping state); and *silence* (representing ultimate reality).

- Sit in a comfortable position.
- Inhale deeply. Exhale and begin chanting the sound of *Om: ah / oh / mmm / silence*.
- Pause. Inhale deeply.
- Chant for 2 more rounds. Increase the volume with each round.
- When you have completed chanting, return your breath to normal and repeat silently:
  My spirit overflows with luminous energy.

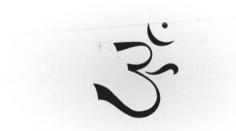

PALMING MEDITATION

Like Walking Meditation (facing page), this meditation uses motion to help calm and soothe. In addition to providing the benefits of other meditations, Palming Meditation diminishes fatigue in the eyes, face, and entire body. It improves concentration and imparts a natural vitality to the eyes. It is a great way to help transition from a hectic day to a quiet evening.

- Sit in any comfortable position with your spine extended. If you wear glasses, remove them and place them nearby. Close your eyes.
- Rub the palms of your hands together vigorously, creating heat and charging them with energy.
- Cup your palms gently over closed eyes, fingers resting lightly on your forehead. Make sure that there is no pressure on your eyeballs.
- Concentrate on relaxing your eyelids and releasing all the tension held in them. Feel the heat of your hands.
- Remain in this position for a minute or more, breathing slowly and deeply as the warmth settles over your eyes.
- Inhale and repeat silently: *I see through new eyes.*
- Exhale and repeat silently: *Beauty is all around me.*
- Bring your hands to the center of your chest in *Namasté* and acknowledge the splendor that surrounds you.
- Lower your arms to your sides. Blink a few times.

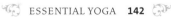

WALKING MEDITATION

You may wish to do this meditation outdoors or in a large room. Stand with your spine comfortably extended and your gaze focused on a spot in front of you. Arms may be by your sides or in front of the heart center in *Namasté*. In addition to offering all the other benefits of meditation, Walking Meditation also increases circulation in the legs and feet.

- Breathe deeply.
- Begin walking by inhaling and raising your right foot. Exhale and place your foot down in front of you.
- Inhale and raise your left foot. Exhale and place your foot down in front of you.
- Take each step slowly and deliberately. Be aware of how you raise your leg. Pay attention to the sensations as you lift your legs and feet up and place them back down.
- Maintain your focus and awareness. Walk as though this was your first time. Nothing else matters, only lifting your foot and placing it back onto the ground.
- Continue at a slow, steady pace. Concentrate on each step and the rhythm of your breath.
- Take a step and repeat silently: *I have no destination.*
- Take the next step and repeat silently: *This is about the journey.*
- Continue until the journey feels complete to you.

SMILING MEDITATION

Studies show that when we smile, we relax hundreds of muscles in our body. A positive message is sent to the mind, and we actually feel calmer, happier, and more at peace.

- Inhale and exhale deeply.
- Inhale and imagine you are breathing in pure, positive energy.
- Exhale slowly, expelling all negativity.
- Continue breathing in this way, inhaling positive energy and exhaling negativity until you feel completely recharged and refreshed.
- Allow a smile to grace your lips.
- Inhale and say: *I feel happy,*
- Exhale and say: *Because I am.*

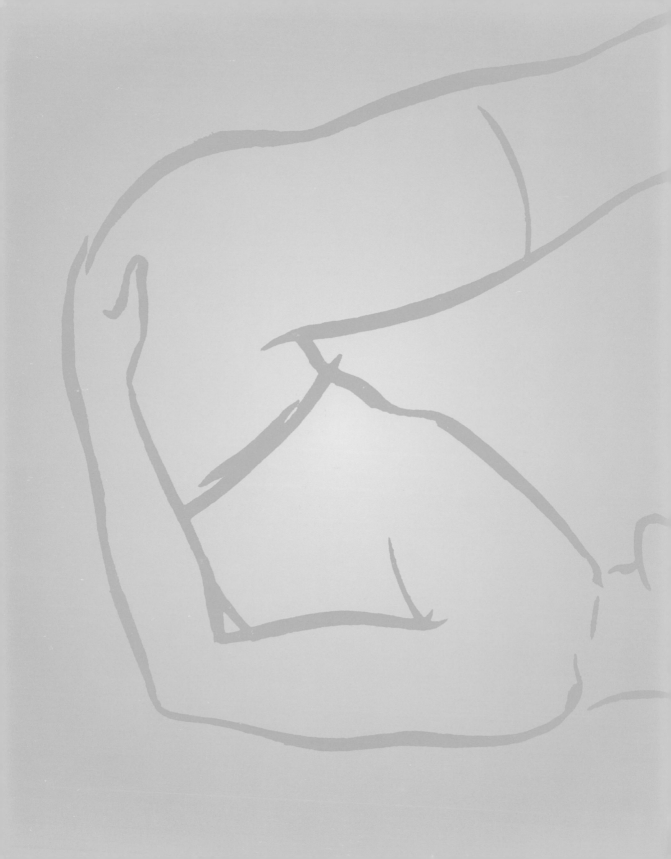

5

FLOWING ROUTINES

LEARNING IS MOVEMENT FROM MOMENT TO MOMENT.
—*J. Krishnamurti*

Yoga poses may be linked together and performed in a particular order as a series (*vinyasa* in Sanskrit). One of the most well-known is Sun Salutation (*Surya Namaskara*), an energetic and dynamic sequence of up to 12 poses. For those who find the full Sun Salutation too challenging or who don't often have time to do the full routine, we have included 2 modifications of Sun Salutation. This chapter also includes Moon Salutation (*Chandra Namaskara*), Camel *vinyasa*, and Energy Stretch *vinyasa*.

Performed like a choreographed dance routine, these sequential yoga poses engage the body, use the breath, and focus the mind. Many people find that once a yoga pose is committed to memory, it becomes easy to add it to a yoga routine. For instance, you may choose to greet each day with *Surya Namaskara* and know that all the muscles throughout your body will be stretched. Complete the day with *Chandra Namaskara* and allow the series of twists and bends to remove all the stiffness and tension from the day.

As you would with every hatha yoga practice, perform the routines with awareness and deliberation. Your breath is an important part of controlling the pace of the movements. Once you are more familiar with a sequence, it will become easier to coordinate the breath and movements. No matter how well you come to know a sequence or how many times you may have performed it, you should never hurry through it in a rote, automatic fashion. However, for a more energetic routine, you may wish to quicken the pace as you flow smoothly and mindfully from one pose to another.

These routines can be quite demanding and strenuous. Please start slowly and make any modifications you need to be comfortable and safe. Don't push beyond your limit. As with any regimen, your strength and stamina will increase as you perform the flowing yoga routines patiently and with persistence and determination.

KNEELING SUN SALUTATION

(*Sidana Surya Namaskara*)

This modification is a good way to build up to the more demanding routine of the full Sun Salutation. The physical movement in synchronicity with the breath provides many of the same benefits without any risk of overexertion.

1. Sit in Thunderbolt pose (page 94). Place your hands in front of your chest in *Namasté*.

2. Inhale and lift your upper body from your buttocks so that you are standing on your knees. Your arms are parallel and raised over your head, palms facing each other. Bend backward slightly so the front of your body gets a slight stretch. Look up at the ceiling, taking care not to overextend your neck.

3. Exhale and bend forward at the hips, coming down onto the floor in Child pose (page 110).

4. Bring elbows in front of you on the floor, palms down. Using your arms, inhale and lift your upper body. Raise your hips and slide the left knee back 5 to 7 inches, followed by the other knee. Slowly lower your upper body onto the floor.

5. Move your arms forward on the floor slightly. Press your pelvis into the floor. Inhale and lift up into Cobra (page 111). Exhale.

6. Curl your toes under, inhale, and on an exhalation, lift into Downward Dog (page 128). Stay for 3 to 5 breaths.

7. Exhale and drop your knees to the floor so your body is in "table position," with your arms under shoulders and knees under hips.

8. Inhale and return to Thunderbolt pose (step 1) with your hands in front of the chest in *Namasté*.

• Repeat the sequence 3 to 4 times.

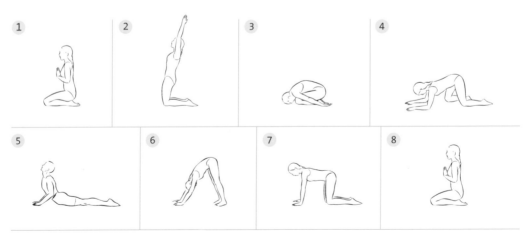

MODIFIED SUN SALUTATION

(Vikrta Surya Namaskara)

This pose is ideal as a warm-up or as a way to gain the strength and flexibility required for the full Sun Salutation. It is also a great way to energize your body when you're tired or when your muscles are stiff after a long day of sitting.

1. Stand in Mountain pose (page 60) with your feet parallel. Place your hands in front of your chest in *Namasté*.

2. Inhale and lift your arms over your head, palms facing but not touching.

3. Exhale and hinge forward at the waist into Forward Bend (page 75); tuck the chin and bend the knees. Palms rest on either side of your feet on the floor; bend your knees if you cannot touch the floor.

4. Inhale and straighten your legs. Engage your abdominal muscles and slowly raise your upper body to an upright position. Exhale. Inhale and lift your hands over your head, with palms facing but not touching. Bend the upper torso back slightly.

5. Exhale and lower your upper body, bending at the waist, back to step 3.

6. Inhale. Engage your abdominal muscles, lift your chin, keeping your knees soft, and return your body to an upright position (step 2). Raise your arms, with palms facing but not touching.

7. Exhale and return to start position with your hands in front of your chest in *Namasté*.

• Repeat 3 to 4 times.

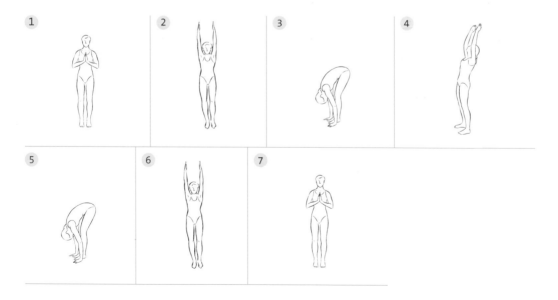

SUN SALUTATION

(Surya Namaskara)

The *ha* of hatha means sun and is associated with dynamic energy, positive force, giving, physical, male, yang, and the right side (*pingala nadi*) of the body. The classic Sun Salutation is a dynamic and beneficial series based on the pose-counterpose system, which alternates between forward-bending and backward-bending postures. It provides aerobic benefits to the cardiovascular system, increasing endurance and warming and energizing the entire system. It expands lung function, increases respiration, and stimulates the body's vital energies. It stretches the spine and improves posture; stretches and strengthens the muscles of the legs, arms, and torso; and improves flexibility. When doing Sun Salutation, give praise to Father Sun, which nourishes and surrounds us with life-giving energy. Let *Surya Namaskara* warm your body and soul.

1 Stand in Mountain pose (page 60) with feet parallel. Keep your hands in front of your chest with palms together in *Namasté*. Inhale and exhale deeply.

2 Inhale and lift your arms over your head, with palms facing but not touching. Bend the upper torso backward slightly.

3 Exhale and bend forward at the waist into Forward Bend (page 75), tucking your chin toward your chest and bending the knees. Your palms rest on either side of your feet on the floor; if you cannot touch the floor, bend your knees slightly.

4 Inhale and extend your left leg straight behind you into Kneeling Lunge (page 86); your knee, shin, and toes rest on the floor. Your right foot is forward between your hands with the knee over the ankle.

5 Exhale and bring your right leg back. Support the weight of your body on your hands and toes. Inhale in a "push-up" position. Your back should be straight, abdominal muscles engaged.

6 Exhale and lower your knees, upper chest, and forehead to the floor. Hips are raised. Hold the breath out for 2 to 3 seconds.

7 Inhale, lower your hips, and raise your upper torso into Cobra (page 111), keeping the shoulders down, pressing the pelvis down into the floor.

8 Exhale and raise your hips into Downward Dog (page 128).

9 Inhale. Step your left foot forward between your hands. Extend your right leg straight behind you; your knee, shin, and toes rest on the floor (step 4 reversed).

10 Exhale, bring the right foot forward, and bend down at the waist, with palms resting on either side of your feet on the floor (step 3). Bend your knees slightly if you cannot touch the floor.

11 Inhale and raise your upper body to an upright position by engaging the abdominals, lifting the chin, and keeping the knees soft (back to step 2). Raise your arms overhead, with palms facing but not touching. Bend the upper body backward slightly.

12 Exhale and return to start position with hands in *Namasté*. Inhale and exhale completely.

• Repeat all 12 steps; this time, bring your right leg backward at step 4.

• Perform *Surya Namaskara* for 3 more rounds if time and energy permit.

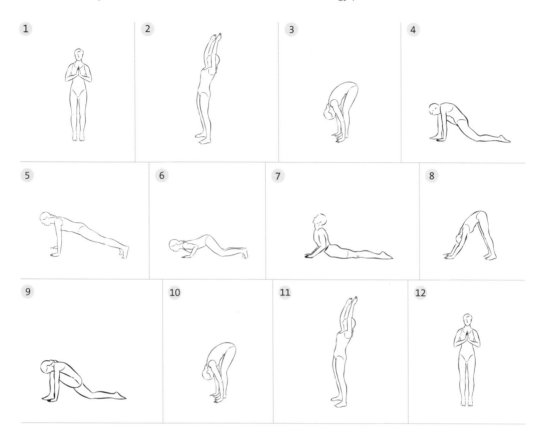

MOON SALUTATION
(*Chandra Namaskara*)

The *tha* of hatha means moon and is associated with static energy, negative force, receiving, spiritual, female, yin, and the left side (*ida nadi*) of the body. Moon Salutation, which is done from a standing position, uses several upper body twists and rotations. This series stretches and tones the muscles along the sides of the body, increases lung capacity and improves respiration, and strengthens the abdominal muscles and arms. It aligns the spinal column and releases tension in the neck, shoulders, and arms. When doing *Chandra Namaskara*, celebrate all of life's mysteries.

1   Stand in Mountain pose (page 60) with your feet a little wider than hip-width apart. Turn your toes out slightly. Palms are together in front of your chest in *Namasté*.

2   Inhale and raise your arms over your head; keep your shoulders down and away from your ears. Separate your arms about 3 feet in a V position; separate your fingers. Raise your head and look up at the ceiling. You are a 5-pointed star.

3   Exhale and separate the feet about 3 feet. Bend both knees and simultaneously bend both elbows at 90°, in Victory Squat (page 74).

4   Inhale and bring the feet closer together under the hips. Raise your arms and clasp your hands overhead. Gaze up at your hands. Don't overextend the neck.

5   Exhale and lower your head. Lower your arms and cross them at the wrists in front of your body.

6   Inhale. Exhale and return to Victory Squat (step 3).

7   Inhale and bring your head back to center and raise your arms to shoulder level, forming a T.

8   Exhale and bend your upper body to the right in Triangle pose (page 63). If you feel strong enough, place your right arm onto your right leg and bend your body farther to the right as far as is comfortable for you.

9   Inhale and return to center, with your arms out to T position (step 7).

10   Exhale and bend your upper body to the left in Triangle Pose (step 8).

11   Inhale and raise your body. Return to center with arms in T position (step 7).

12   Exhale and bring your hands together in front of your chest, palms together in *Namasté*.

•   Repeat once more on both sides.

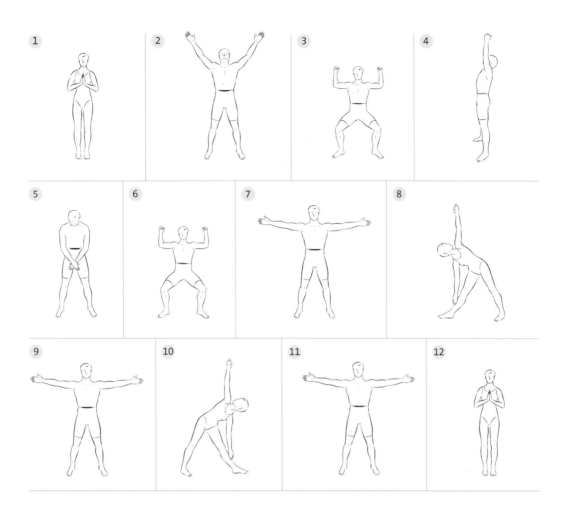

CAMEL VINYASA
(*Kubahula Vinyasa*)

Camel *vinyasa* opens the chest and strengthens the upper thigh muscles and the muscles along the back. This series tones the buttocks and stretches the arms, neck, throat, and front of the thighs. It also stimulates the abdominal organs and increases circulation and energy flow. If steps 11 and 12 are too intense at first, repeat step 8 instead. This is a very demanding routine. Individuals with lower back problems should consult a yoga instructor before attempting Camel *vinyasa*. Those with high blood pressure or a herniated disk should not do this series.

1   Begin in Thunderbolt (page 94). Place a folded blanket either across your calf muscles or under the backs of your knees.

2   Inhale and raise your buttocks from your heels. Lift your arms overhead, and interlace the fingers with palms turned up.

3   Exhale and bend your elbows so your interlaced fingers come behind your neck. Remain in the pose for several breaths: Inhale, allowing your chest to lift up; exhale, soften, and relax.

4   Inhale and raise your arms again. With your fingers still interlaced, turn your hands so your palms face down.

5   Exhale and bend at the waist in Child pose (page 110) with arms extended on the floor in front of you.

6   Inhale and bring your hands onto your lower back, with palms facing up. Engage your abdominal muscles firmly and attempt to keep your buttocks on your heels as you raise your upper body back to Thunderbolt (step 1).

7   Exhale and bring your hands to the floor behind you, about a foot away from your body. Keep your palms flat on the floor, with fingers pointing toward your body. Your body should be leaning back at a slight angle, your head aligned with the spine.

8   Inhale and press your pelvis forward in a modified Camel pose (page 88). Imagine that you are pressing the front of your body against a wall. Hold for 2 to 3 breaths.

9   Exhale and lower your hips, going back to step 7.

10   Return to Child pose (step 5).

11   Inhale and raise your upper body to a kneeling position. Your arms hang by your sides, and your shoulders are down and away from your ears.

12   Exhale, consciously engage the abdominal muscles, and slowly reach back with your hands, grasping your heels in Camel pose (page 88). If this is too difficult, curl your toes under and hold onto your raised heels. Inhale and, keeping your abdominal muscles active, press your pelvis

forward as you lift your chest and drop your head back slightly. Take care not to overextend your neck. Hold for 2 to 3 breaths.

13 Inhale, and one at a time, release your hands from your heels, and straighten your upper body (step 11).

14 Exhale and lower your buttocks onto your heels in Thunderbolt pose (step 1).

15 Rest in Child pose for 30 seconds to 1 minute (step 5), with your arms extended on the floor in front of you, palms down, or by your sides with palms up.

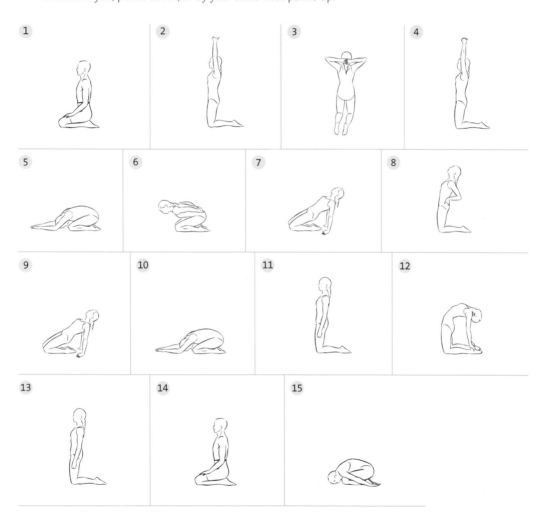

ENERGY-STRETCH VINYASA

(Shakti Uttana Vinyasa)

This series stimulates and rebalances the flow of energy throughout the body. It increases flexibility and stretches the muscles of the legs, chest, and shoulders. It also aligns the spine and opens the hips. For the seated poses, you may sit on a folded blanket or towel to maintain the normal curve in the lower back. Do not allow your back to round in the seated postures.

1 Sit with your spine comfortably extended, shoulders down and away from your ears. Inhale and bend your legs, bringing the soles of your feet together in Bound Angle (page 100). Grasp your feet with your hands. Exhale and bend forward, hinging at your hips as you maintain an extended spine. Sitting bones keep sinking into the mat or folded blanket. If you can, lower your chin towards the floor. Hold for 5 deep breaths. Inhale and return to an upright position.

2 Sit on the floor with your spine comfortably extended. Place both legs straight on the floor in front of you, separated comfortably. Your toes and knees point up. Exhale and grasp your feet with both hands in Seated Angle (page 100). Lower your upper body until you feel your back begin to round. Stop, maintaining an extension of the spine. Feel the breastbone extending away from the navel. Hold for 8 to 12 breaths. Inhale and return to an upright position.

3 Sit with your spine comfortably extended, shoulders down and away from your ears. Your legs are straight on the floor in front of you, your feet together. Inhale and hinge forward from the waist, lowering your chest toward your thighs. Grasp your feet with both hands in Sitting Forward Bend (page 103). Bend your knees if the stretch becomes too intense. Hold for a complete breath and return to an upright position.

4 Sit in Easy pose (page 90) with your spine comfortably extended. Rest your right hand on your left knee and your left hand on your right knee.

5 Exhale and bend forward from the waist, extending the breastbone away from your navel. Keep the sitting bones in contact with the floor and bend forward with the intention of resting your forehead on the floor. Breathe deeply. Inhale and return to an upright position.

6 Stand with your feet separated a little wider than your shoulders. Inhale and lift your arms over your head, with fingers interlaced. Bend your upper body to the right in Half Moon pose (page 62) as far as you can. Breathe deeply. Inhale and return to center. Repeat on the opposite side. Alternate twice on each side.

7 Stand with your feet about shoulder-width apart. Clasp your hands behind your back, exhale, and bend forward from the waist in Yoga Mudra (page 77). Let your arms fall forward as far as you can; let your head hang loosely. Hold on to a strap with both hands if the shoulders are tight. Breathe. Inhale and return to an upright position. Repeat Yoga Mudra once more.

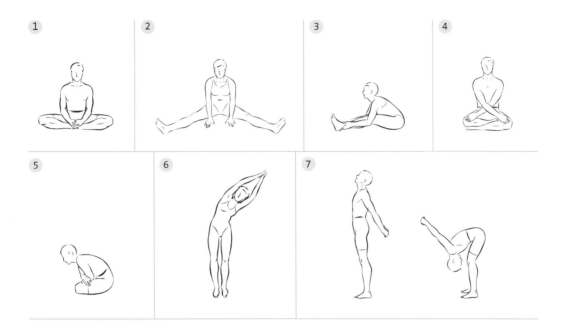

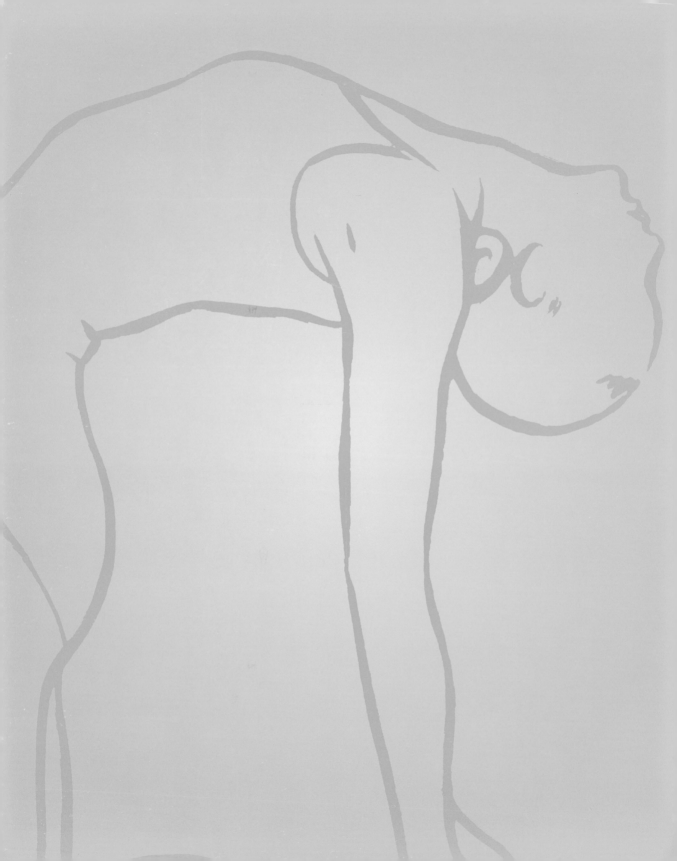

6

YOGA SESSIONS

THE BODY IS MORTAL, BUT THE PERSON DWELLING IN THE BODY
IS IMMORTAL AND IMMEASURABLE.

—*Bhagavad Gita*

The following yoga sessions are suggested to help you incorporate yoga into your routine. Remember that they are recommendations only. Make any changes, additions, or substitutions that you wish. If time permits, add a meditation of your choice or a moment of relaxation after the sequence. You may also wish to close your session with an additional breathing exercise. Please note that the times given are approximate and meant as general guidelines.

Note: When a pose works one side of the body and then the other, don't forget to repeat the pose on the opposite side.

MORNING SESSION (35 TO 45 MINUTES):

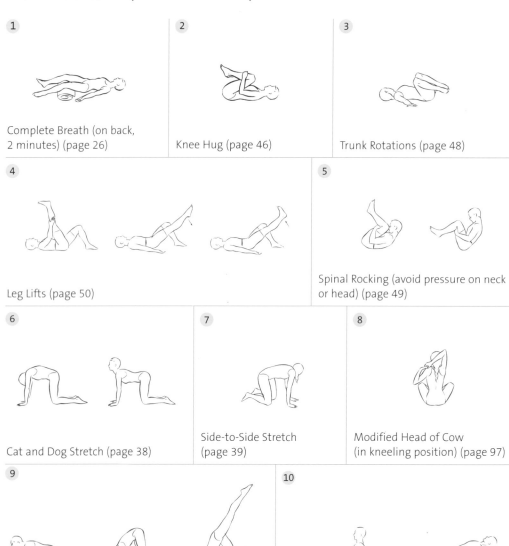

1

Complete Breath (on back, 2 minutes) (page 26)

2

Knee Hug (page 46)

3

Trunk Rotations (page 48)

4

Leg Lifts (page 50)

5

Spinal Rocking (avoid pressure on neck or head) (page 49)

6

Cat and Dog Stretch (page 38)

7

Side-to-Side Stretch (page 39)

8

Modified Head of Cow (in kneeling position) (page 97)

9

Downward Dog (page 128)

10

Inclined Plane (page 109)

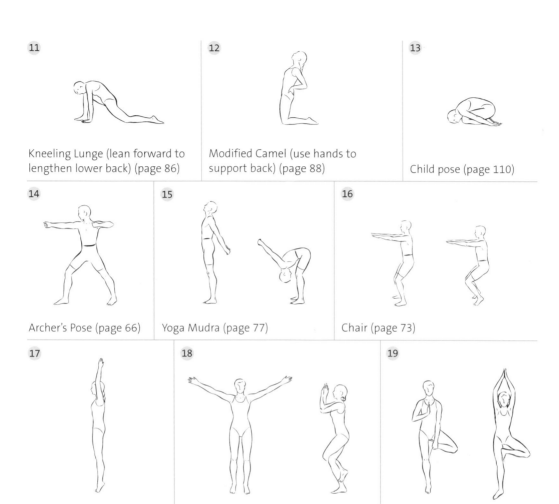

11 Kneeling Lunge (lean forward to lengthen lower back) (page 86)

12 Modified Camel (use hands to support back) (page 88)

13 Child pose (page 110)

14 Archer's Pose (page 66)

15 Yoga Mudra (page 77)

16 Chair (page 73)

17 Standing-on-Toes (page 61)

18 Eagle (page 72)

19 Tree (page 70)

20

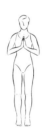

Mountain (rest for 2 to 3 minutes, silently repeating a phrase or mantra or focusing on your breath) (page 60)

EVENING SESSION (25 TO 30 MINUTES):

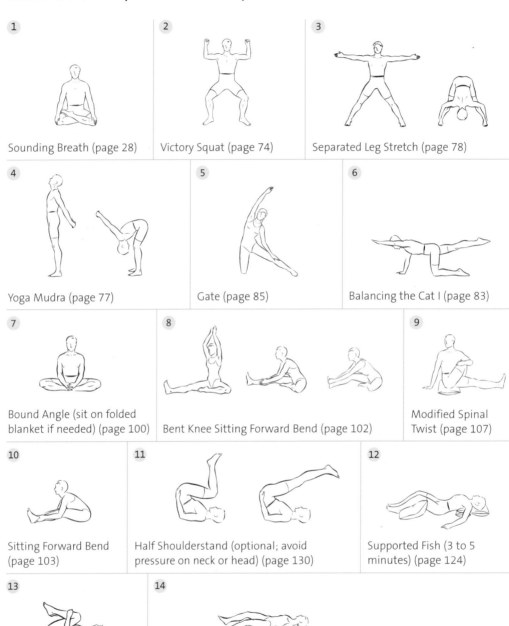

1 Sounding Breath (page 28)

2 Victory Squat (page 74)

3 Separated Leg Stretch (page 78)

4 Yoga Mudra (page 77)

5 Gate (page 85)

6 Balancing the Cat I (page 83)

7 Bound Angle (sit on folded blanket if needed) (page 100)

8 Bent Knee Sitting Forward Bend (page 102)

9 Modified Spinal Twist (page 107)

10 Sitting Forward Bend (page 103)

11 Half Shoulderstand (optional; avoid pressure on neck or head) (page 130)

12 Supported Fish (3 to 5 minutes) (page 124)

13 Knee Hug (page 46)

14 Corpse (up to 5 minutes; place thick rolled blanket[s] under knees) (page 127)

LOWER BACK PROBLEMS (20 TO 30 MINUTES):

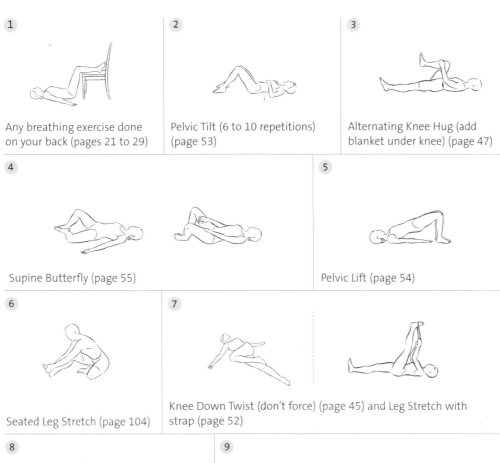

1 Any breathing exercise done on your back (pages 21 to 29)

2 Pelvic Tilt (6 to 10 repetitions) (page 53)

3 Alternating Knee Hug (add blanket under knee) (page 47)

4 Supine Butterfly (page 55)

5 Pelvic Lift (page 54)

6 Seated Leg Stretch (page 104)

7 Knee Down Twist (don't force) (page 45) and Leg Stretch with strap (page 52)

8 Through-the-Hole Stretch (page 119)

9 Cat and Dog Stretch (page 38)

Lower Back Problems continued on page 162 ▶ ▶ ▶

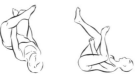 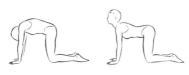

▶ ▶ ▶ *Lower Back Problems continued from page 161*

10

Balancing the Cat I (page 83)

11

Sphinx (page 56) or Cobra as back becomes stronger (page 111)

12

Half Locust (page 115)

13

Child pose (page 110)

14

Reclining Spinal Twist (page 122)

15

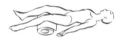

Corpse (up to 10 minutes; place thick rolled blanket[s] under knees) (page 127)

GENERAL SESSION (45 MINUTES TO 1 HOUR):

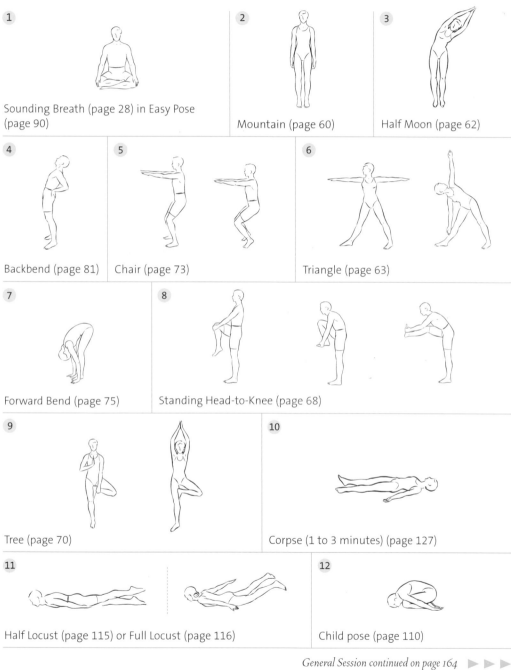

1 Sounding Breath (page 28) in Easy Pose (page 90)

2 Mountain (page 60)

3 Half Moon (page 62)

4 Backbend (page 81)

5 Chair (page 73)

6 Triangle (page 63)

7 Forward Bend (page 75)

8 Standing Head-to-Knee (page 68)

9 Tree (page 70)

10 Corpse (1 to 3 minutes) (page 127)

11 Half Locust (page 115) or Full Locust (page 116)

12 Child pose (page 110)

General Session continued on page 164 ▶ ▶ ▶

▶ ▶ ▶ *General Session continued from page 163*

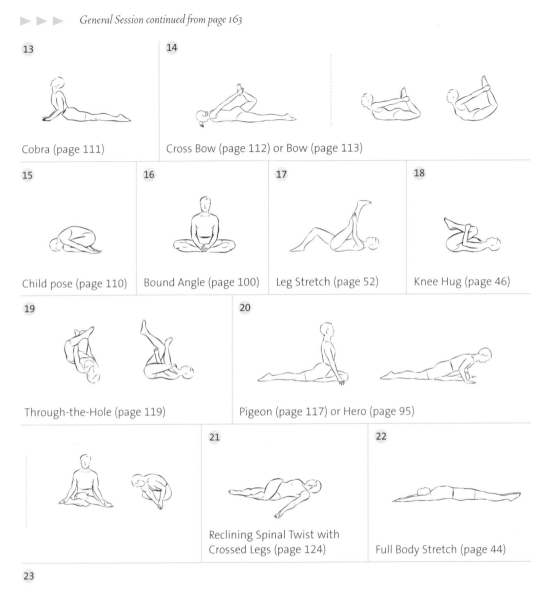

13

Cobra (page 111)

14

Cross Bow (page 112) or Bow (page 113)

15

Child pose (page 110)

16

Bound Angle (page 100)

17

Leg Stretch (page 52)

18

Knee Hug (page 46)

19

Through-the-Hole (page 119)

20

Pigeon (page 117) or Hero (page 95)

21

Reclining Spinal Twist with Crossed Legs (page 124)

22

Full Body Stretch (page 44)

23

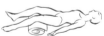

Corpse (10 minutes or longer; place thick rolled blanket[s] under knees) (page 127)

GENERAL SESSION I (1 HOUR):

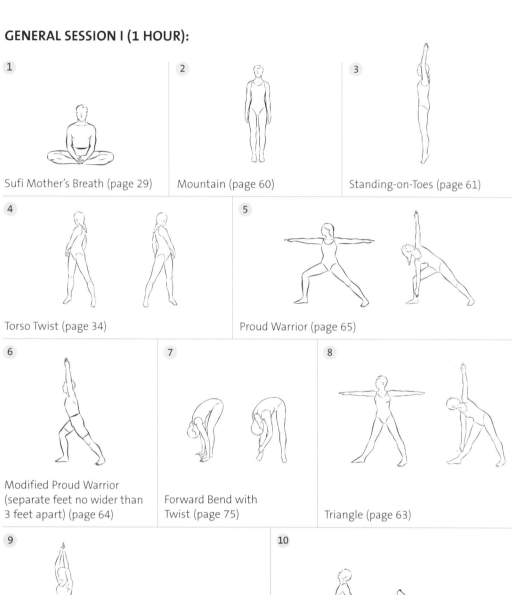

1 Sufi Mother's Breath (page 29)

2 Mountain (page 60)

3 Standing-on-Toes (page 61)

4 Torso Twist (page 34)

5 Proud Warrior (page 65)

6 Modified Proud Warrior (separate feet no wider than 3 feet apart) (page 64)

7 Forward Bend with Twist (page 75)

8 Triangle (page 63)

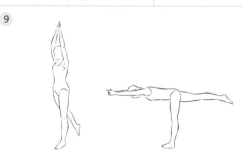

9 Balancing Stick (using a chair is optional) (page 71)

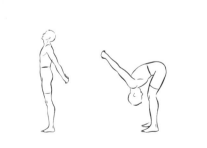

10 Yoga Mudra (page 77)

General Session I continued on page 166 ▶ ▶ ▶

► ► ► *General Session I continued from page 165*

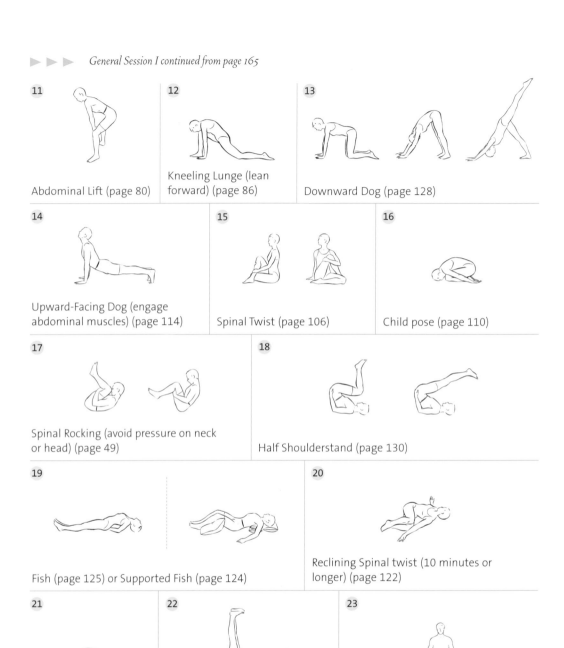

11 Abdominal Lift (page 80)

12 Kneeling Lunge (lean forward) (page 86)

13 Downward Dog (page 128)

14 Upward-Facing Dog (engage abdominal muscles) (page 114)

15 Spinal Twist (page 106)

16 Child pose (page 110)

17 Spinal Rocking (avoid pressure on neck or head) (page 49)

18 Half Shoulderstand (page 130)

19 Fish (page 125) or Supported Fish (page 124)

20 Reclining Spinal twist (10 minutes or longer) (page 122)

21 Child pose (page 110)

22 Legs-Against-Wall (page 133)

23 Any meditation (5 minutes or longer) (pages 136 to 143)

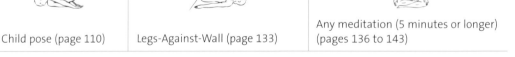

GENERAL SESSION II (1 HOUR):

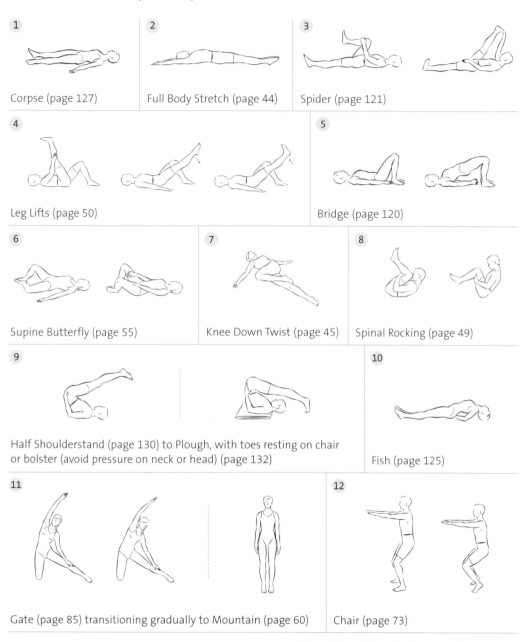

1 Corpse (page 127)

2 Full Body Stretch (page 44)

3 Spider (page 121)

4 Leg Lifts (page 50)

5 Bridge (page 120)

6 Supine Butterfly (page 55)

7 Knee Down Twist (page 45)

8 Spinal Rocking (page 49)

9 Half Shoulderstand (page 130) to Plough, with toes resting on chair or bolster (avoid pressure on neck or head) (page 132)

10 Fish (page 125)

11 Gate (page 85) transitioning gradually to Mountain (page 60)

12 Chair (page 73)

General Session II continued on page 168 ▶ ▶ ▶

▶ ▶ ▶ *General Session II continued from page 167*

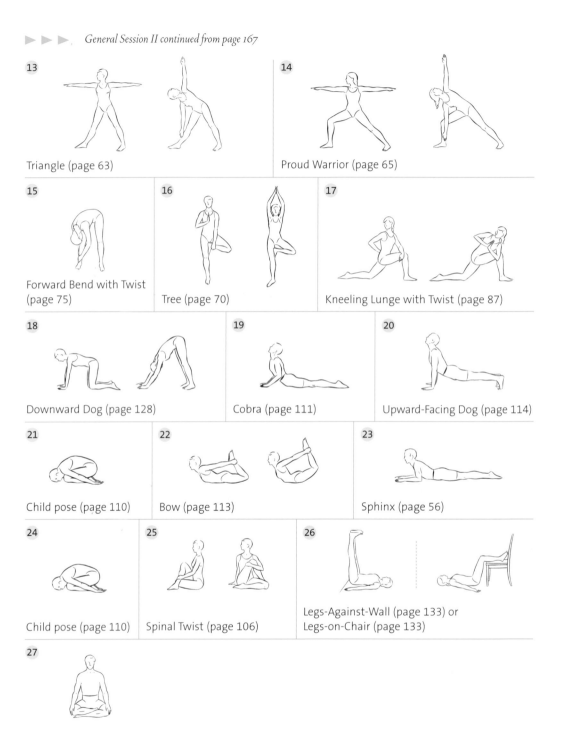

13
Triangle (page 63)

14
Proud Warrior (page 65)

15
Forward Bend with Twist (page 75)

16
Tree (page 70)

17
Kneeling Lunge with Twist (page 87)

18
Downward Dog (page 128)

19
Cobra (page 111)

20
Upward-Facing Dog (page 114)

21
Child pose (page 110)

22
Bow (page 113)

23
Sphinx (page 56)

24
Child pose (page 110)

25
Spinal Twist (page 106)

26
Legs-Against-Wall (page 133) or Legs-on-Chair (page 133)

27
Any seated meditation (10 minutes) (pages 137 to 142)

GENERAL SESSION (1 TO 1½ HOURS):

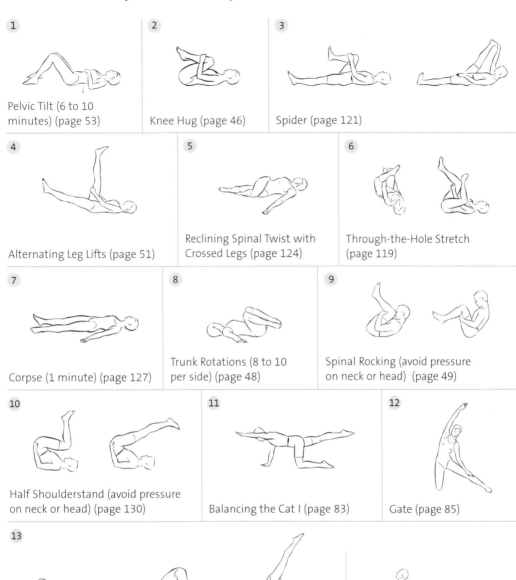

1 Pelvic Tilt (6 to 10 minutes) (page 53)

2 Knee Hug (page 46)

3 Spider (page 121)

4 Alternating Leg Lifts (page 51)

5 Reclining Spinal Twist with Crossed Legs (page 124)

6 Through-the-Hole Stretch (page 119)

7 Corpse (1 minute) (page 127)

8 Trunk Rotations (8 to 10 per side) (page 48)

9 Spinal Rocking (avoid pressure on neck or head) (page 49)

10 Half Shoulderstand (avoid pressure on neck or head) (page 130)

11 Balancing the Cat I (page 83)

12 Gate (page 85)

13 Downward Dog (page 128) to Upward-Facing Dog (page 114)

General Session continued on page 170 ▶ ▶ ▶

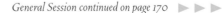

▶ ▶ ▶ *General Session continued from page 169*

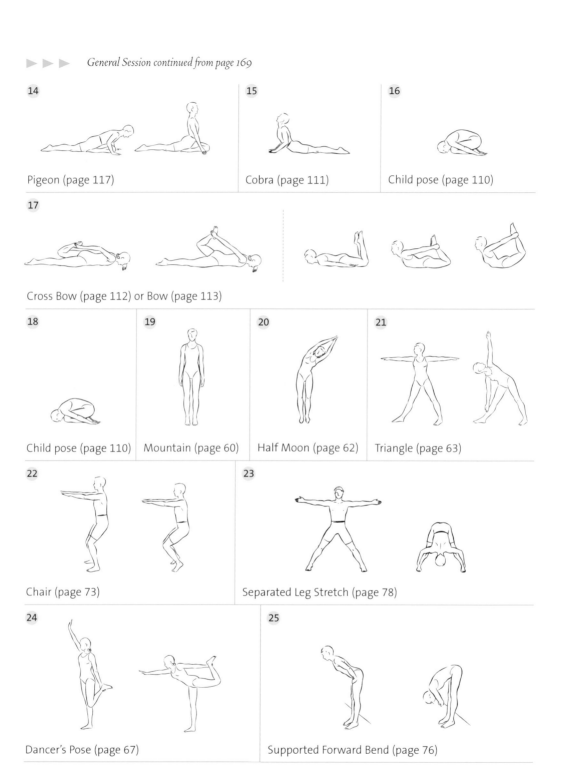

14 Pigeon (page 117)

15 Cobra (page 111)

16 Child pose (page 110)

17 Cross Bow (page 112) or Bow (page 113)

18 Child pose (page 110)

19 Mountain (page 60)

20 Half Moon (page 62)

21 Triangle (page 63)

22 Chair (page 73)

23 Separated Leg Stretch (page 78)

24 Dancer's Pose (page 67)

25 Supported Forward Bend (page 76)

26

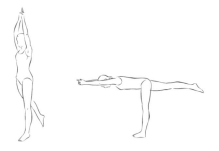

Balancing Stick (page 71)

27

Standing Side Stretch (page 69)

28

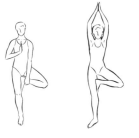

Tree (page 70)

29

Hero (add gentle seated spinal twist) (page 95)

30

Reclining Spinal Twist with Extended Legs (page 123)

31

Knee Hug (page 46)

32

Corpse (10 minutes or longer; place thick rolled blanket[s] under the knees) (page 127)

INVERTED SESSION (1 HOUR)

This sequence is recommended for yoga practitioners with supple spines, without lower back or neck issues, and without high blood pressure, glaucoma, or other issues related to the eyes.

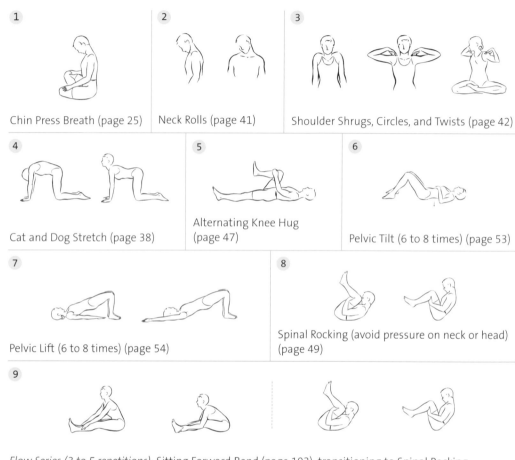

1. Chin Press Breath (page 25)
2. Neck Rolls (page 41)
3. Shoulder Shrugs, Circles, and Twists (page 42)
4. Cat and Dog Stretch (page 38)
5. Alternating Knee Hug (page 47)
6. Pelvic Tilt (6 to 8 times) (page 53)
7. Pelvic Lift (6 to 8 times) (page 54)
8. Spinal Rocking (avoid pressure on neck or head) (page 49)
9.

Flow Series (3 to 5 repetitions): Sitting Forward Bend (page 103), transitioning to Spinal Rocking (avoid pressure on neck or head) (page 49) . . .

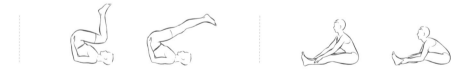

. . . into a Half Shoulderstand (page 130). Pause and lower spine down gradually, placing hands on the floor beyond the buttocks. Engage abdominals and come into Sitting Forward Bend (page 103).

10

Flow Series (3 to 5 repetitions): Sitting Forward Bend (page 103), transitioning to Spinal Rocking (page 49), into Plough, with toes resting on chair or bolster (page 132) . . .

. . . lowering down to Sitting Forward Bend (page 103).

11

Bridge (page 120)

12

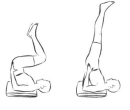

Full Shoulderstand (avoid pressure on neck or head) (page 131)

13

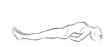

Fish (page 125)

14

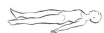

Corpse (up to 10 minutes) (page 127)

15

Any seated meditation (pages 137 to 142)

DYNAMIC SESSION (1½ HOURS):

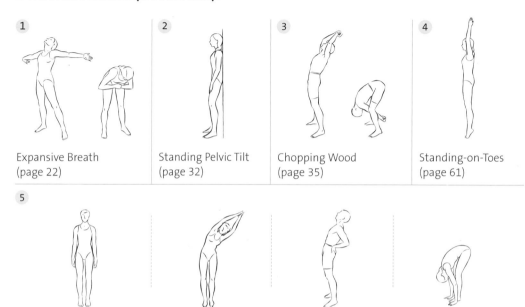

1 Expansive Breath (page 22)

2 Standing Pelvic Tilt (page 32)

3 Chopping Wood (page 35)

4 Standing-on-Toes (page 61)

5

Flow Series (2 repetitions): Mountain (page 60), to Half Moon (page 62), to Backbend (with hands supporting lower back) (page 81), to Forward Bend (hands slide down to back of thighs and calves, coming around to the front) (page 75)

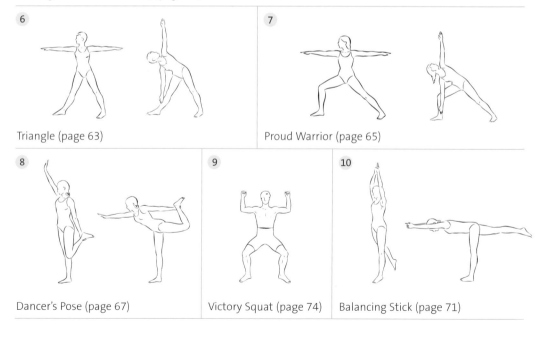

6 Triangle (page 63)

7 Proud Warrior (page 65)

8 Dancer's Pose (page 67)

9 Victory Squat (page 74)

10 Balancing Stick (page 71)

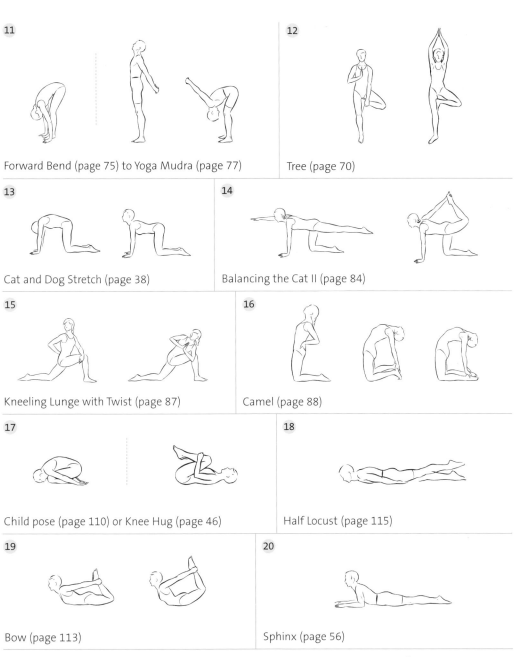

11

Forward Bend (page 75) to Yoga Mudra (page 77)

12

Tree (page 70)

13

Cat and Dog Stretch (page 38)

14

Balancing the Cat II (page 84)

15

Kneeling Lunge with Twist (page 87)

16

Camel (page 88)

17

Child pose (page 110) or Knee Hug (page 46)

18

Half Locust (page 115)

19

Bow (page 113)

20

Sphinx (page 56)

Dynamic Session continued on page 176 ▶ ▶ ▶

► ► ► *Dynamic Session continued from page 175*

21

Child pose (page 110) or Knee Hug (page 46)

22

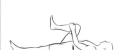

Spider (page 121)

23

Bound Angle (page 100)

24

Knee Rocking (page 101)

25

Seated Head-to-Knee (page 105)

26

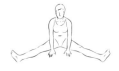

Seated Angle (page 100)

27

Alternate Nostril Breath (page 21) while seated in Half Lotus (page 90) (up to 2 minutes)

28

Finish by sitting quietly, allowing your breath to be soft and soothing (up to 10 minutes)

PREPARATION FOR SUN SALUTATION (1½ HOURS):

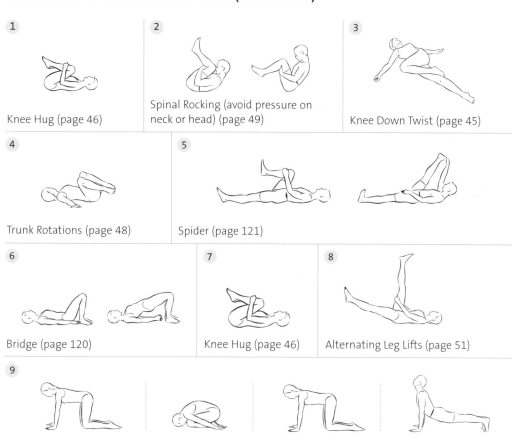

1 Knee Hug (page 46)

2 Spinal Rocking (avoid pressure on neck or head) (page 49)

3 Knee Down Twist (page 45)

4 Trunk Rotations (page 48)

5 Spider (page 121)

6 Bridge (page 120)

7 Knee Hug (page 46)

8 Alternating Leg Lifts (page 51)

9

Flow Series (3 repetitions): Begin in Table Position (page 38). Exhale and bring hips back toward heels in Child pose (page 110). Inhale back into Table Position (page 38), then up into Upward-Facing Dog (page 114).

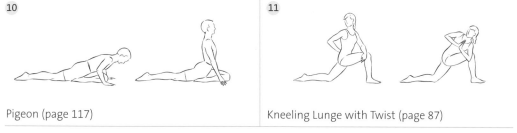

10 Pigeon (page 117)

11 Kneeling Lunge with Twist (page 87)

Preparation for Sun Salutation continued on page 178 ▶ ▶ ▶

▶ ▶ ▶ *Preparation for Sun Salutation continued from page 177*

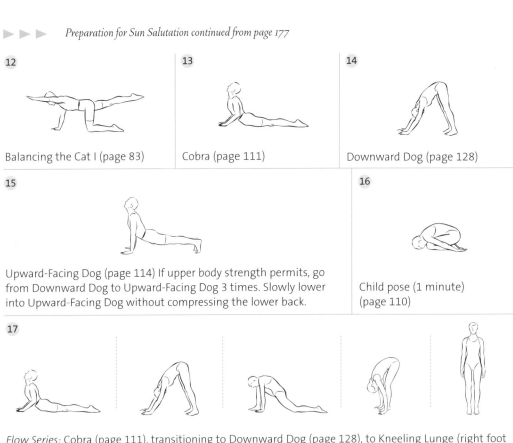

12 Balancing the Cat I (page 83)

13 Cobra (page 111)

14 Downward Dog (page 128)

15 Upward-Facing Dog (page 114) If upper body strength permits, go from Downward Dog to Upward-Facing Dog 3 times. Slowly lower into Upward-Facing Dog without compressing the lower back.

16 Child pose (1 minute) (page 110)

17 *Flow Series:* Cobra (page 111), transitioning to Downward Dog (page 128), to Kneeling Lunge (right foot forward) (page 86), to Forward Bend (page 75), to Mountain (page 60). Repeat, bringing left foot forward.

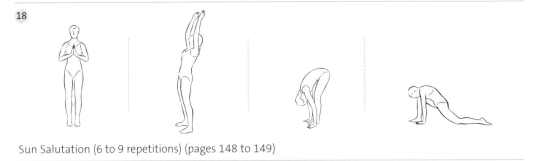

18 Sun Salutation (6 to 9 repetitions) (pages 148 to 149)

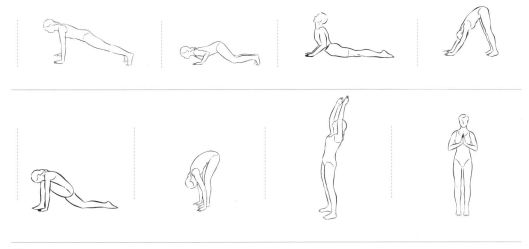

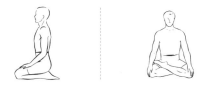

Finish in Thunderbolt (page 94) or Half Lotus (page 90) (5 to 10 minutes), performing a breathing exercise of your choice (pages 21 to 29). Add another layer of clothing to stay warm.

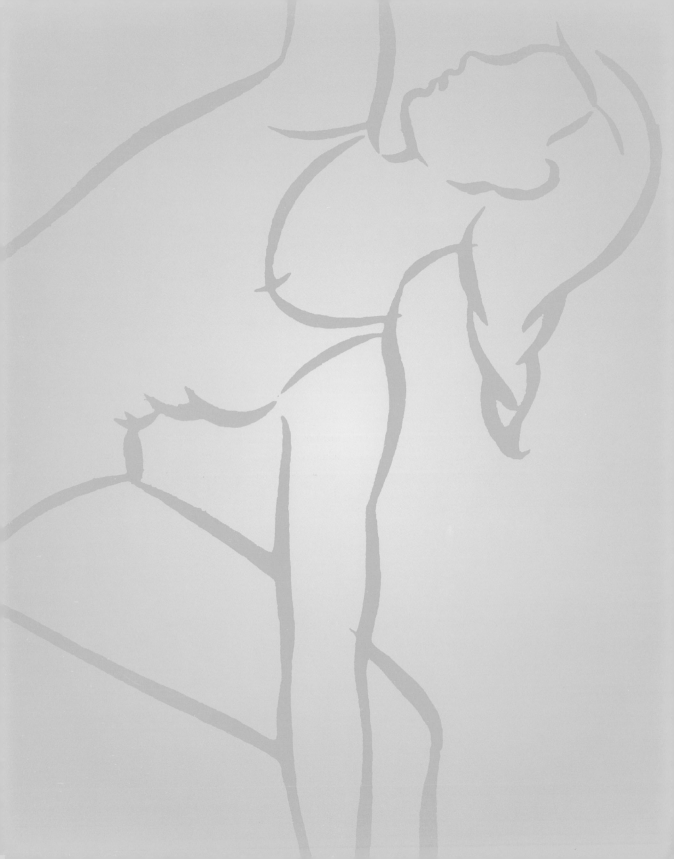

7

RECOMMENDED SEQUENCES

AND THE END OF ALL OUR EXPLORING
WILL BE TO ARRIVE WHERE WE STARTED
AND TO KNOW THE PLACE FOR THE FIRST TIME.
—T. S. ELIOT

The following forty-eight 10 to 15 minute sequences are included as simple, targeted programs. Some help alleviate various conditions such as anxiety, tension, hip discomfort, and back pain. Others focus on improving overall health with sessions designed to help prevent colds, boost energy levels, and strengthen the body. In addition, we have included sessions to help prepare for specific activities such as biking, dancing, racquet sports, and golfing. As with the sessions in chapter 6, remember to repeat poses that work one side of the body on the opposite side.

ALL-OVER STRETCH

1

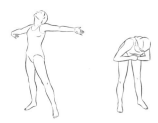

Expansive Breath (page 22)

2

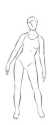 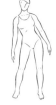

Barrel Movement (page 33)

3

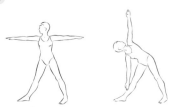

Triangle (page 63)

4

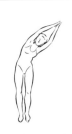

Half Moon (page 62)

5

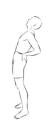

Backbend (page 81)

6

Forward Bend with Twist (page 75)

7

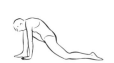

Kneeling Lunge (page 86)

8

Bound Angle (page 100)

9

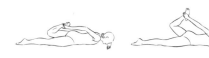

Cross Bow (page 112)

10

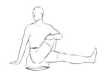

Modified Spinal Twist (page 107) or Reclining Spinal Twist (page 122)

ANXIETY/TENSION RELIEF

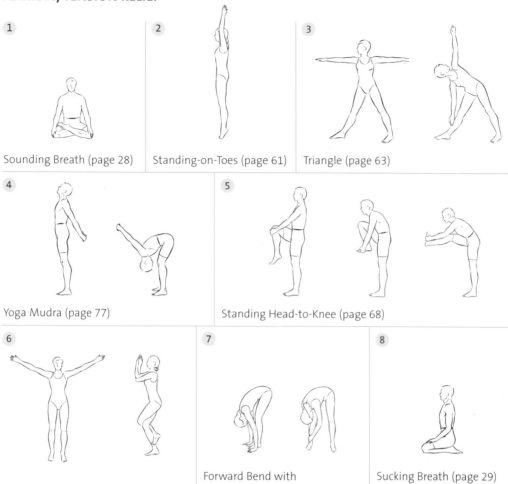

1 Sounding Breath (page 28)

2 Standing-on-Toes (page 61)

3 Triangle (page 63)

4 Yoga Mudra (page 77)

5 Standing Head-to-Knee (page 68)

6 Eagle (page 72)

7 Forward Bend with Twist (page 75)

8 Sucking Breath (page 29) in Thunderbolt (page 94)

BACK PAIN RELIEF

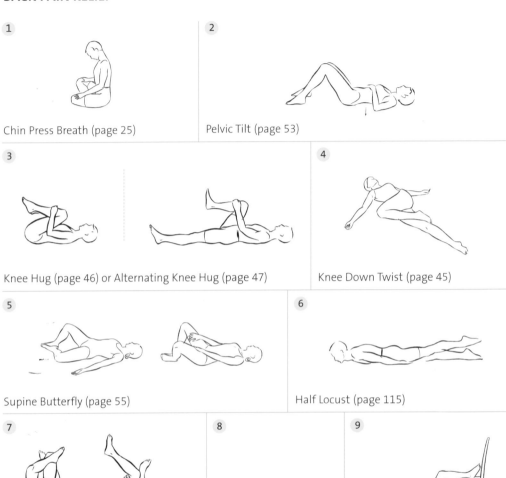

1 Chin Press Breath (page 25)

2 Pelvic Tilt (page 53)

3 Knee Hug (page 46) or Alternating Knee Hug (page 47)

4 Knee Down Twist (page 45)

5 Supine Butterfly (page 55)

6 Half Locust (page 115)

7 Through-the-Hole Stretch (page 119)

8 Child pose (page 110)

9 Legs-on-Chair (page 133)

BALANCE AND CONCENTRATION

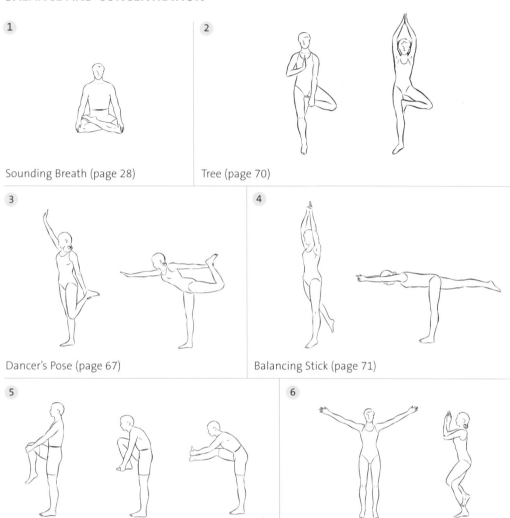

1 Sounding Breath (page 28)

2 Tree (page 70)

3 Dancer's Pose (page 67)

4 Balancing Stick (page 71)

5 Standing Head-to-Knee (page 68)

6 Eagle (page 72)

COMPLEXION (FOUNTAIN OF YOUTH)

1

Complete Breath (page 26)

2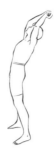

Chopping Wood (page 35)

3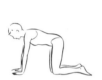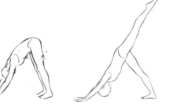

Downward Dog (page 128)

4

Kneeling Yoga Mudra (page 82)

5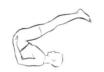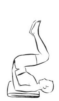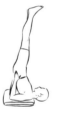

Half (page 130) or Full Shoulderstand (avoid pressure on neck or head) (page 131)

6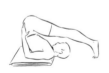

Plough (page 132)

7

Lion (page 98)

COLD PREVENTION

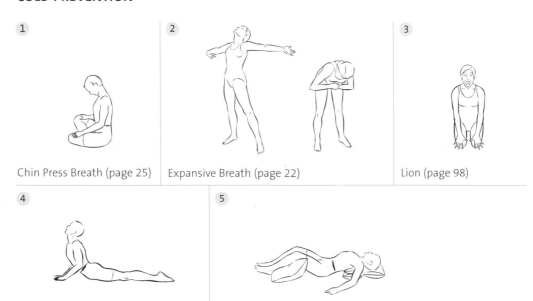

1. Chin Press Breath (page 25)

2. Expansive Breath (page 22)

3. Lion (page 98)

4. Cobra (page 111)

5. Supported Fish (page 124)

DEPRESSION RELIEF

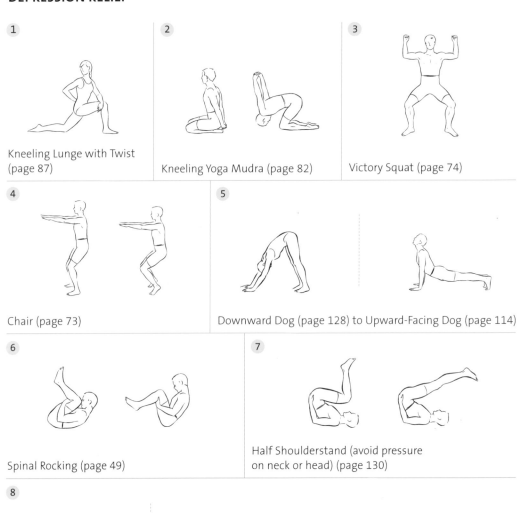

1 Kneeling Lunge with Twist (page 87)

2 Kneeling Yoga Mudra (page 82)

3 Victory Squat (page 74)

4 Chair (page 73)

5 Downward Dog (page 128) to Upward-Facing Dog (page 114)

6 Spinal Rocking (page 49)

7 Half Shoulderstand (avoid pressure on neck or head) (page 130)

8 Fish (page 125) or Supported Fish (page 124)

ENERGY BOOST

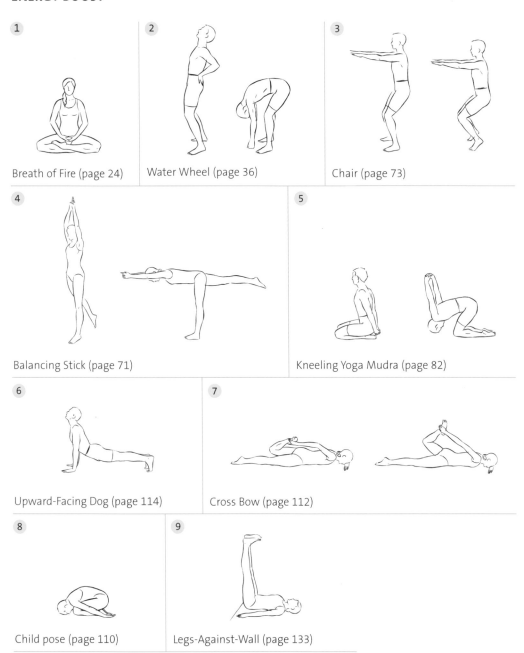

1 Breath of Fire (page 24)

2 Water Wheel (page 36)

3 Chair (page 73)

4 Balancing Stick (page 71)

5 Kneeling Yoga Mudra (page 82)

6 Upward-Facing Dog (page 114)

7 Cross Bow (page 112)

8 Child pose (page 110)

9 Legs-Against-Wall (page 133)

FLEXIBILITY

1

Any breathing exercise
(pages 21 to 29)

2

Neck Rolls (page 41)

3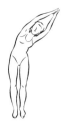

Half Moon (page 62)

4

Kneeling Lunge with Twist (page 87)

5

Half Locust (page 115)

6

Through-the-Hole Stretch
(page 119)

7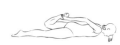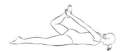

Bow (page 113) or Cross Bow (page 112)

8

Sitting Forward Bend (page 103)

HEADACHE/EYE STRAIN RELIEF

1

Alternate Nostril Breath (page 21)

2

Neck Rolls (page 41)

3

 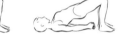

Shoulder Shrugs, Circles, and Twists (page 42)

4

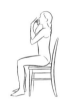

Blade (page 43)

5

Bridge (page 120)

6

Seated Eagle (page 93)

7

Lion (page 98)

8

Sounding Breath (page 28) performed in Easy Pose (page 90)

9

Palming Meditation (page 142)

HIP DISCOMFORT RELIEF

1

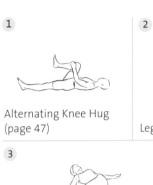

Alternating Knee Hug
(page 47)

2

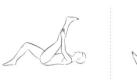 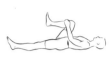 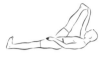

Leg Stretch (page 52) or Spider (page 121)

3

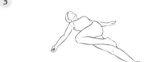

Knee Down Twist (page 45)

4

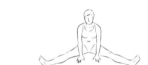

Supine Butterfly (page 55)

5

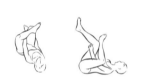 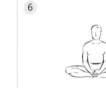

Through-the-Hole Stretch (page 119)

6

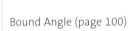

Bound Angle (page 100)

7

Seated Angle (page 100)

8

Reclining Spinal Twist
(page 122)

9

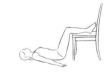

Legs-on-Chair (page 133) while performing
Sounding Breath (page 28)

IMMUNE SYSTEM BOOST

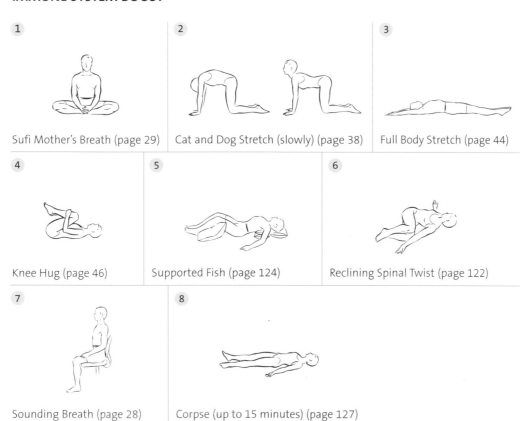

1. Sufi Mother's Breath (page 29)

2. Cat and Dog Stretch (slowly) (page 38)

3. Full Body Stretch (page 44)

4. Knee Hug (page 46)

5. Supported Fish (page 124)

6. Reclining Spinal Twist (page 122)

7. Sounding Breath (page 28)

8. Corpse (up to 15 minutes) (page 127)

IMPROVING CIRCULATION

   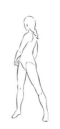 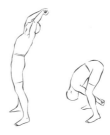

Breath of Fire with Raised Thumbs (page 24) or Expansive Breath (page 22)

Torso Twist (page 34)

Chopping Wood (page 35)

 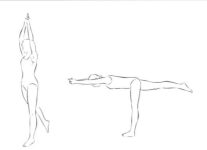   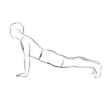

Balancing Stick (page 71)

Downward Dog (page 128) to Upward-Facing Dog (3 to 6 repetitions) (page 114)

 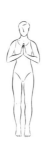 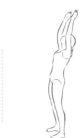 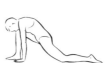

Sun Salutation (page 148)

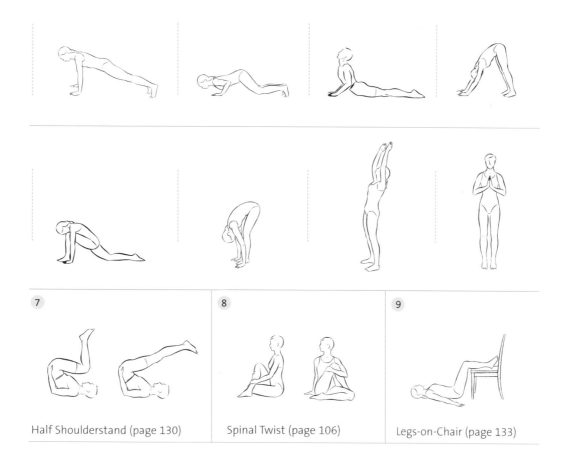

7 Half Shoulderstand (page 130)

8 Spinal Twist (page 106)

9 Legs-on-Chair (page 133)

KNEE STRENGTHENER

1

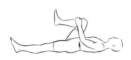

Alternating Knee Hug (page 47)

2

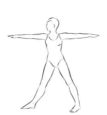
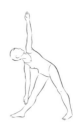

Triangle (make sure that knee, shinbone, and ankle are aligned) (page 63)

3

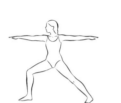
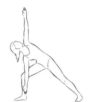

Proud Warrior (ensure that bent knee is directly over ankle) (page 65)

4

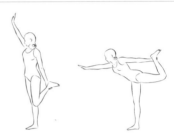

Dancer's Pose (feel lifting of kneecap on standing leg) (page 67)

5

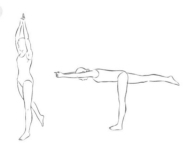

Balancing Stick (strengthens quadriceps) (page 71)

6

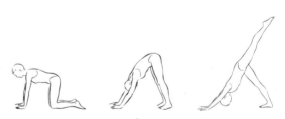

Downward Dog (feet hip distance apart, keeping knee properly aligned) (page 128)

7

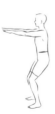
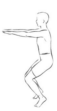

Chair (separate feet a little more than hip distance, keeping thighs and shins absolutely parallel to protect knees) (page 73)

MENSTRUAL CRAMPS RELIEF

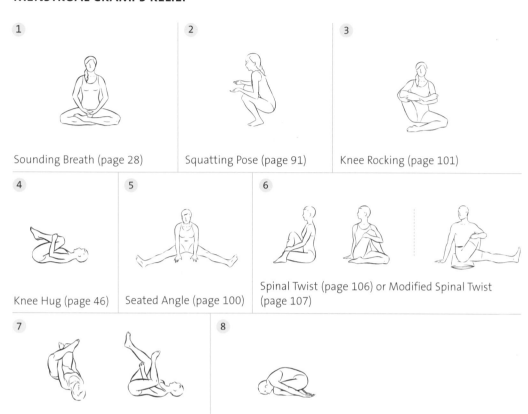

1 Sounding Breath (page 28)

2 Squatting Pose (page 91)

3 Knee Rocking (page 101)

4 Knee Hug (page 46)

5 Seated Angle (page 100)

6 Spinal Twist (page 106) or Modified Spinal Twist (page 107)

7 Through-the-Hole Stretch (page 119)

8 Child pose (page 110)

MENTAL FATIGUE RELIEF

1

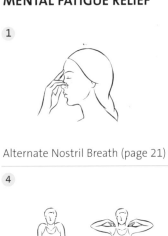

Alternate Nostril Breath (page 21)

2

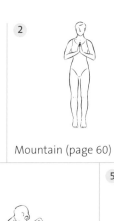

Mountain (page 60)

3

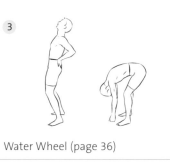

Water Wheel (page 36)

4

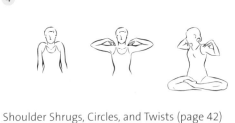

Shoulder Shrugs, Circles, and Twists (page 42)

5

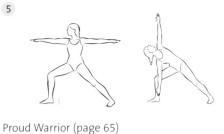

Proud Warrior (page 65)

6

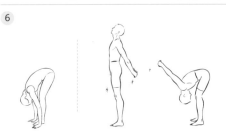

Forward Bend (page 75) to Yoga Mudra (slowly) (page 77)

7

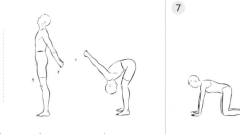

Downward Dog (page 128)

8

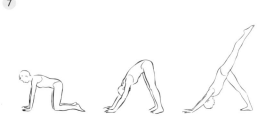

Half Shoulderstand (page 130)

9

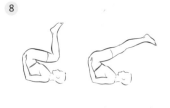

Sounding Breath (page 28)

10

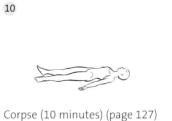

Corpse (10 minutes) (page 127)

MOOD ENHANCERS

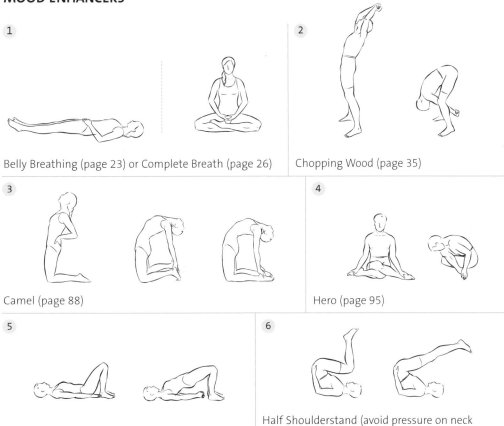

1 Belly Breathing (page 23) or Complete Breath (page 26)

2 Chopping Wood (page 35)

3 Camel (page 88)

4 Hero (page 95)

5 Bridge (page 120)

6 Half Shoulderstand (avoid pressure on neck or head) (page 130)

7

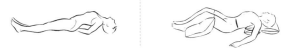

Fish (page 125) or Supported Fish (page 124)

OVER 60

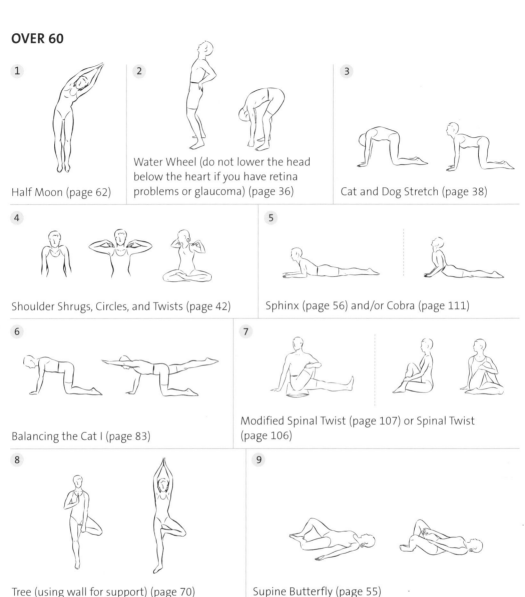

1 Half Moon (page 62)

2 Water Wheel (do not lower the head below the heart if you have retina problems or glaucoma) (page 36)

3 Cat and Dog Stretch (page 38)

4 Shoulder Shrugs, Circles, and Twists (page 42)

5 Sphinx (page 56) and/or Cobra (page 111)

6 Balancing the Cat I (page 83)

7 Modified Spinal Twist (page 107) or Spinal Twist (page 106)

8 Tree (using wall for support) (page 70)

9 Supine Butterfly (page 55)

10 Knee Down Twist (page 45)

11 Sounding Breath (page 28) while in Legs-on-Chair (page 133)

PRENATAL

1

Belly and Chest Breathing (page 23)

2

Blade (page 43)

3

Modified Head of Cow (page 97)

4

Cat and Dog Stretch (page 38)

5

Standing Pelvic Tilt (page 32)

6

Backbend (page 81)

7

Walking Meditation (page 143)

RELAXATION AND STRESS RELIEF

1

Humming Bee Breath (page 27)

2

Neck Rolls (page 41)

3

Knee Hug (page 46) or Alternating Knee Hug (page 47)

4

Reclining Spinal Twist (page 122)

5

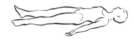

Corpse (15 minutes) (page 127)

RESPIRATORY AILMENTS RELIEF

1

Complete Breath (if possible) (page 26)

2

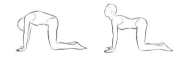

Cat and Dog Stretch (slowly) (page 38)

3

Side-to-Side Stretch (page 39)

4

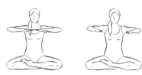

Blade (page 43)

5

Modified Head of Cow (page 97)

6

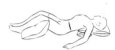

Supported Fish (page 124)

7

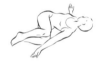

Reclining Spinal Twist (page 122)

8

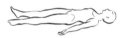

Corpse (up to 15 minutes) (page 127)

SCIATICA RELIEF

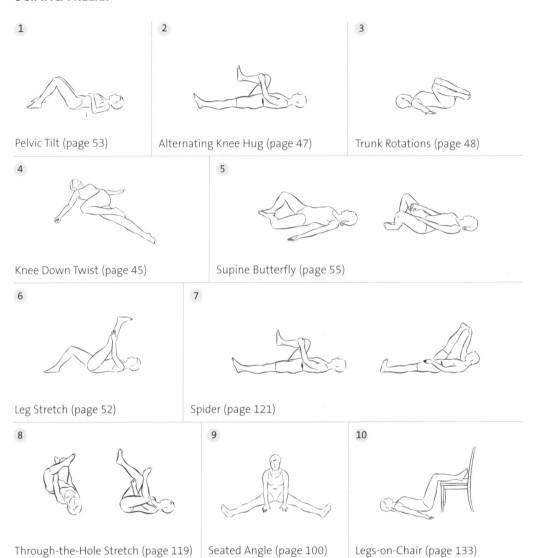

1 Pelvic Tilt (page 53)

2 Alternating Knee Hug (page 47)

3 Trunk Rotations (page 48)

4 Knee Down Twist (page 45)

5 Supine Butterfly (page 55)

6 Leg Stretch (page 52)

7 Spider (page 121)

8 Through-the-Hole Stretch (page 119)

9 Seated Angle (page 100)

10 Legs-on-Chair (page 133)

STRENGTH

1

Breath of Fire with Raised Thumbs (page 24)

2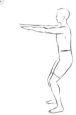

Chair (page 73)

3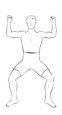

Victory Squat (page 74)

4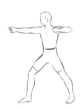

Archer's Pose (page 66)

5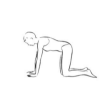

Downward Dog (page 128)

6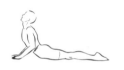

Cobra (page 111)

7

Boat (page 108)

TOXIN FLUSH

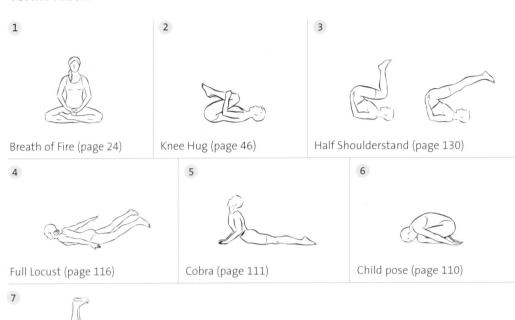

1 Breath of Fire (page 24)

2 Knee Hug (page 46)

3 Half Shoulderstand (page 130)

4 Full Locust (page 116)

5 Cobra (page 111)

6 Child pose (page 110)

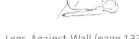

7 Legs-Against-Wall (page 133)

UPPER BACK/NECK PAIN RELIEF

1

Complete Breath (page 26)

2

Shoulder Shrugs, Circles, and Twists (page 42)

3

Torso Twists (page 34)

4

 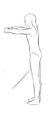

Hands-to-Wall Stretch (page 37)

5

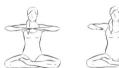

Blade (page 43)

6

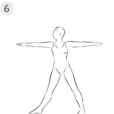 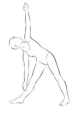

Triangle (page 63)

7

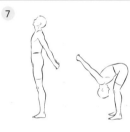

Yoga Mudra (page 77)

8

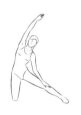

Gate (page 85)

9

Modified Head of Cow (page 97)

RELIEF FOR VARICOSE VEINS

1

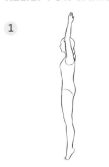

Standing-on-Toes (page 61)

2

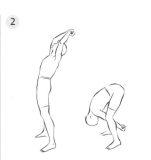

Chopping Wood (page 35)

3

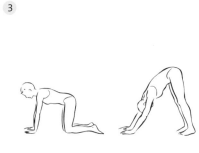

Downward Dog (page 128)

4

  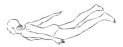

Bow (page 113) or Full Locust (page 116)

5

Knee Hug (page 46)

6

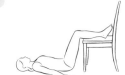

Half Shoulderstand (avoid pressure on neck or head) (page 130)

7

Legs-on-Chair (page 133)

WAKE-UP POSES

1

Breath of Fire with Raised
Thumbs (page 24)

2

Neck Rolls (page 41)

3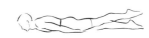

Half Locust (page 115)

4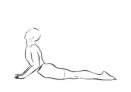

Cobra (page 111)

5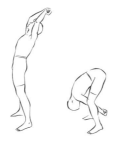

Chopping Wood (page 35)

6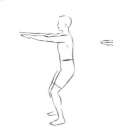

Chair (page 73)

7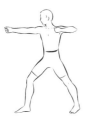

Archer's Pose (page 66)

WEIGHT-BEARING SEQUENCE

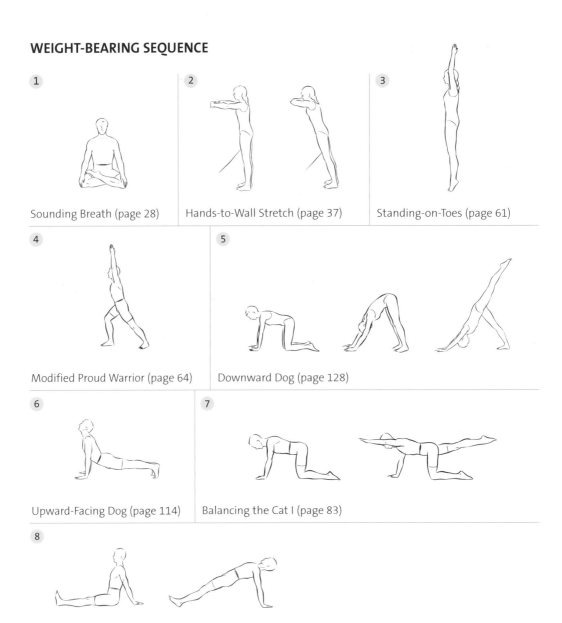

1 Sounding Breath (page 28)

2 Hands-to-Wall Stretch (page 37)

3 Standing-on-Toes (page 61)

4 Modified Proud Warrior (page 64)

5 Downward Dog (page 128)

6 Upward-Facing Dog (page 114)

7 Balancing the Cat I (page 83)

8 Inclined Plane (page 109)

WINDING DOWN POSES

1

Sufi Mother's Breath (page 29)

2

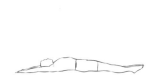

Full Body Stretch (page 44)

3

Thunderbolt (page 94)

4

Seated Eagle (page 93)

5

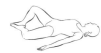

Supine Butterfly (page 55)

6

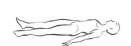

Corpse (5 minutes)
(page 127)

7

Any meditation (pages 137 to 143)

For Specific Activities

(10 to 15 minutes each)

BICYCLING

1

Breath of Fire (page 24)

2

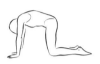

Cat and Dog Stretch (page 38)

3

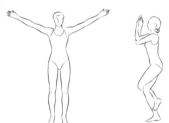

Eagle (page 72)

4

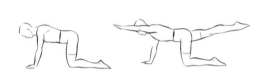

Balancing the Cat I (page 83)

5

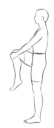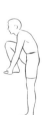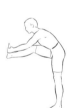

Standing Head-to-Knee (page 68)

6

Reclining Spinal Twist with Extended Legs (page 123)

7

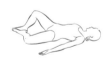

Supine Butterfly (page 55)

BODY WORK

1

Alternate Nostril Breath (page 21)

2

Shoulder Shrugs, Circles, and Twists (page 42)

3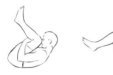

Spinal Rocking (page 49)

4

Modified Head of Cow (page 97) or Head of Cow (page 96)

5

Kneeling Yoga Mudra (page 82)

6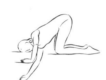

Threading the Needle (page 40)

7

Legs-Against-Wall (page 133)

DANCING

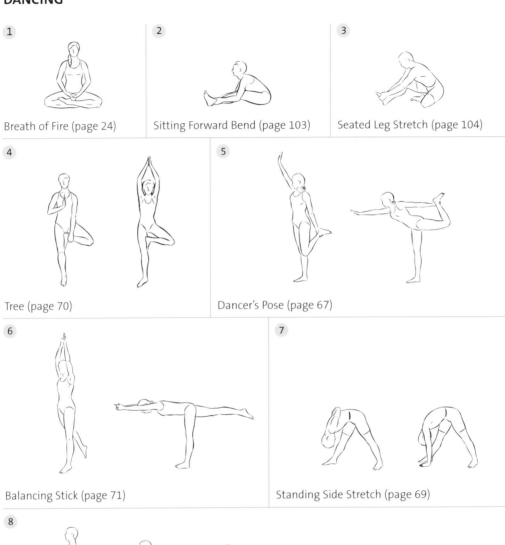

1 Breath of Fire (page 24)

2 Sitting Forward Bend (page 103)

3 Seated Leg Stretch (page 104)

4 Tree (page 70)

5 Dancer's Pose (page 67)

6 Balancing Stick (page 71)

7 Standing Side Stretch (page 69)

8 Standing Head-to-Knee (page 68)

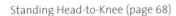

FUN WITH KIDS

 1 **2** 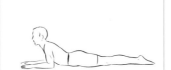 **3**

Humming Bee Breath (page 27)   Sphinx (page 56)   Windshield Wiper Legs (page 57)

4   **5** 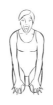   **6**

Modified Head of Cow (page 97)   Lion (page 98)   Turtle (page 99)

7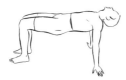

Crab (page 126)

GOLFING

1

Any breathing exercise (pages 21 to 29)

2

Torso Twist (page 34)

3

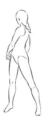

Shoulder Shrugs, Circles, and Twists (from standing position) (page 42)

4

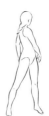

Yoga Mudra (page 77)

5

Head of Cow (from standing position) (page 96)

6

Backbend (page 81)

7

Half Moon (page 62) or Triangle (page 63)

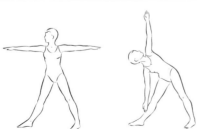

8

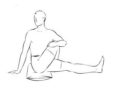

Modified Spinal Twist (page 107)

HIKING

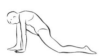

Any breathing exercise
(pages 21 to 29)

Alternating Knee Hug
(page 47)

Standing-on-Toes
(page 61)

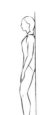

Standing Pelvic Tilt
(page 32)

Kneeling Lunge (page 86)

Through-the-Hole Stretch (page 119)

OFFICE WORK

 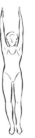 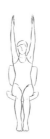

Complete Breath (page 26)

Mountain (page 60) or Seated Mountain (page 92)

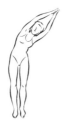 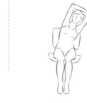

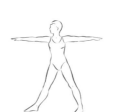 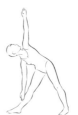

Half Moon (page 62) or Seated Half Moon (page 92)

Triangle (page 63)

Head of Cow (page 96) or Modified Head of Cow (page 97)

Spinal Twist (page 106)

RACQUET SPORTS

1

Any breathing exercise (pages 21 to 29)

2

Shoulder Shrugs, Circles, and Twists (page 42)

3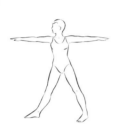

Triangle (page 63)

4

Dancer's Pose (page 67)

5

Squatting Pose (page 91)

6

Upward-Facing Dog (page 114)

7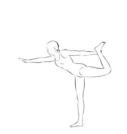

Pelvic Lift (page 54)

8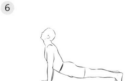

Bridge (page 120)

9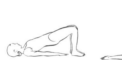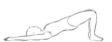

Knee Hug (page 46) or Alternating Knee Hug (page 47)

10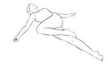

Knee Down Twist (don't force; don't go beyond
stacking one hip over the other) (page 45)

ROWING

1

Complete Breath (page 26)

2

Neck Rolls (page 41)

3

Shoulder Shrugs, Circles, and Twists (page 42)

4

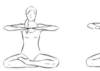

Blade (page 43)

5

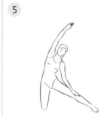

Gate (page 85)

6

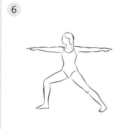

Proud Warrior (page 65)

7

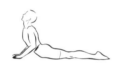

Cobra (page 111)

8

Child pose (page 110)

RUNNING

  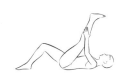 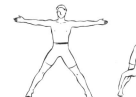

1 Any breathing exercise (pages 21 to 29)

2 Leg Stretch (page 52)

3 Separated Leg Stretch (page 78)

4 Forward Bend (page 75), Forward Bend with Twist (page 75), or Supported Forward Bend (page 76)

5 Knee Rocking (page 101)

 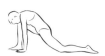

6 Bound Angle (page 100)

7 Kneeling Lunge (page 86)

SKIING

Humming Bee Breath (page 27)

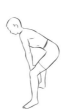

Abdominal Lift (page 80)

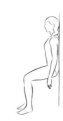

Bent Knee Pelvic Tilt (page 79)

 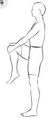 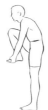 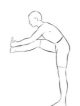

Standing Head-to-Knee (page 68)

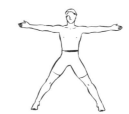

Separated Leg Stretch (page 78)

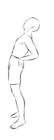

Backbend (page 81)

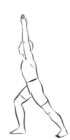

Modified Proud Warrior (page 64)

SWIMMING

1

Complete Breath (page 26)

2

Shoulder Shrugs, Circles, and Twists (page 42)

3

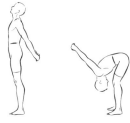

Yoga Mudra (page 77)

4

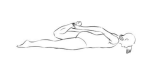

Cross Bow (page 112)

5

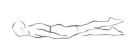

Half Locust (page 115) or Full Locust (page 116)

6

Bridge (page 120)

7

Child pose (page 110)

TENNIS

1

Shoulder Shrugs, Circles, and Twists (from standing position) (page 42)

2

Blade (from standing position) (page 43)

3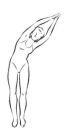

Half Moon (page 62)

4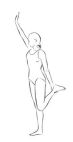

Dancer's Pose (page 67)

5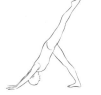

Downward Dog (page 128)

6

Spinal Twist (page 106)

7

Trunk Rotations (page 48)

8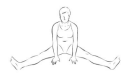

Seated Angle (page 100)

TRAVELING AND COMMUTING

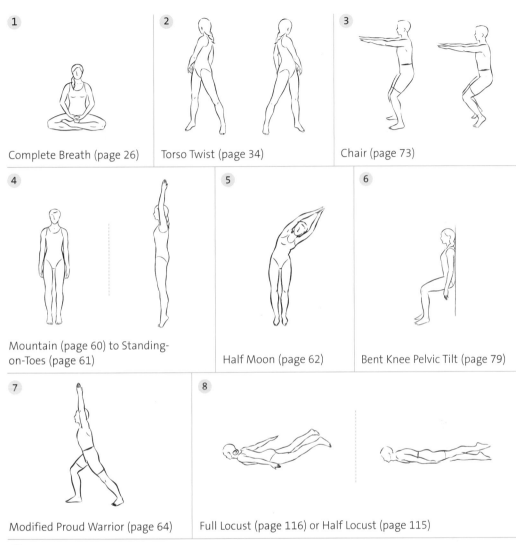

1 Complete Breath (page 26)

2 Torso Twist (page 34)

3 Chair (page 73)

4 Mountain (page 60) to Standing-on-Toes (page 61)

5 Half Moon (page 62)

6 Bent Knee Pelvic Tilt (page 79)

7 Modified Proud Warrior (page 64)

8 Full Locust (page 116) or Half Locust (page 115)

9 Bridge (page 120)

WEIGHT TRAINING

1

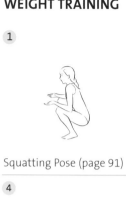

Squatting Pose (page 91)

2

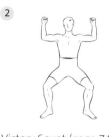

Victory Squat (page 74)

3

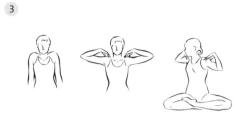

Shoulder Shrugs, Circles, and Twists (page 42)

4

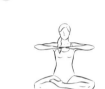

Blade (page 43)

5

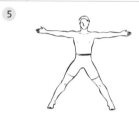

Separated Leg Stretch (page 78)

6

Yoga Mudra (page 77)

7

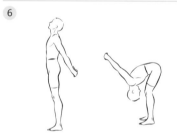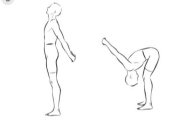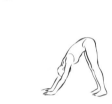

Downward Dog (page 128) to Upward-Facing Dog (page 114)

8

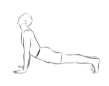

Spinal Twist (page 106)

AUTHOR'S FAVORITES

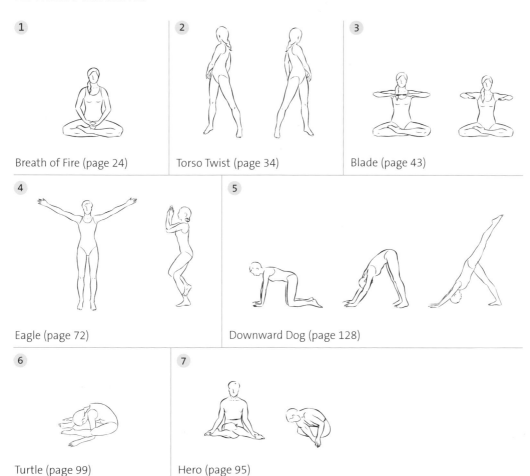

1. Breath of Fire (page 24)

2. Torso Twist (page 34)

3. Blade (page 43)

4. Eagle (page 72)

5. Downward Dog (page 128)

6. Turtle (page 99)

7. Hero (page 95)

YOGA CONSULTANT'S FAVORITES

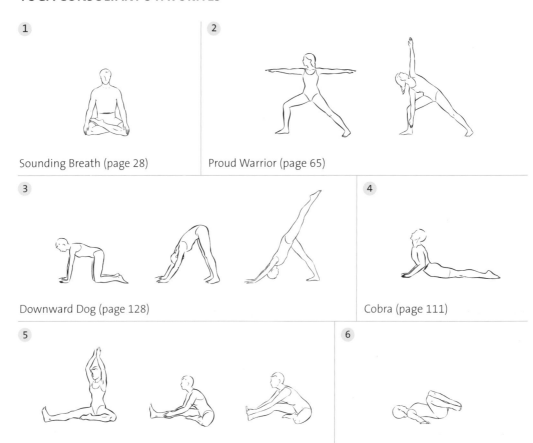

1 Sounding Breath (page 28)

2 Proud Warrior (page 65)

3 Downward Dog (page 128)

4 Cobra (page 111)

5 Bent Knee Sitting Forward Bend (page 102)

6 Trunk Rotations (page 48)

TOP-10 ESSENTIAL YOGA POSES

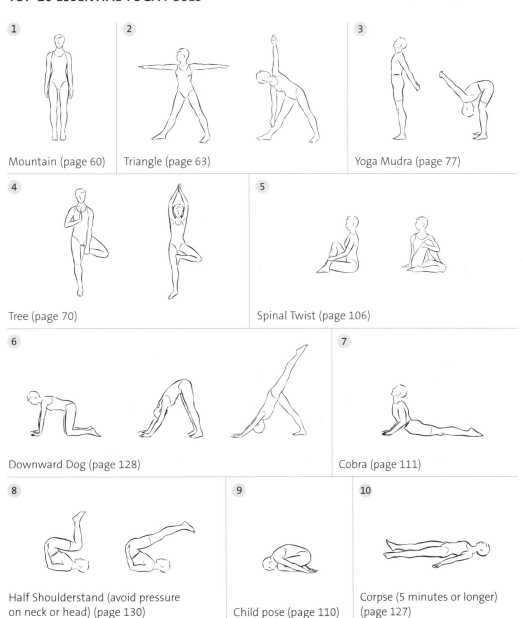

Mountain (page 60)

Triangle (page 63)

Yoga Mudra (page 77)

Tree (page 70)

Spinal Twist (page 106)

Downward Dog (page 128)

Cobra (page 111)

Half Shoulderstand (avoid pressure on neck or head) (page 130)

Child pose (page 110)

Corpse (5 minutes or longer) (page 127)

DON'T JUST SIT THERE, DO YOGA!

Knee Rocking (while putting on socks) (page 101)

Complete Breath (page 26) in Mountain (while waiting in line) (page 60)

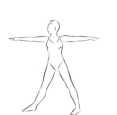
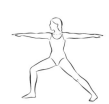
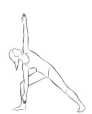

Triangle (page 63) or Proud Warrior (while booting up the computer) (page 65)

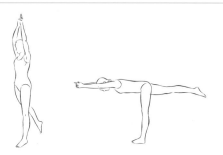

Balancing Stick (while waiting for water to boil) (page 71)

Bound Angle (while watching TV) (page 100)

REFERENCES

There are countless books, organizations, and Web sites out there related to yoga. Here are a few of the more useful ones to get you started.

Books

Choudhury, Bikram. *Bikram's Beginning Yoga Class*. New York: HarperCollins, 2003.

Christensen, Alice. *Yoga of the Heart*. Emmaus, PA: Rodale Press, 1998.

Desikachar, T.K.V. *The Heart of Yoga: Developing a Personal Practice*. Rochester, VT: Inner Traditions, 1995.

Feuerstein, Georg. *The Shambhala Encyclopedia of Yoga*. Boston: Shambhala Publications, 1997.

Feuerstein, Georg. *The Shambhala Guide to Yoga*. Boston: Shambhala Publications, 1996.

Feuerstein, Georg. *The Yoga Tradition: Its History, Religion, Philosophy and Practice*. Prescott, AZ: Holm Press, 2001.

Iyengar, B.K.S. *Light on Yoga*. New York: Shcocken Books, 1979.

Iyengar, B. K. S. *Yoga: The Path to Holistic Health*. London: Doring Kindersley, 2001.

Iyengar, B.K.S. *Tree of Yoga*. Boston: Shambhala Publications, 1984.

Kraftsow, Gary. *Yoga for Transformation: Ancient Teachings and Practices for Healing the Body, Mind, and Heart*. New York: Penguin, 2002.

Lasater, Judith. *Relax and Renew: Restful Yoga for Stressful Times*. Berkeley, CA: Rodmell Press, 1995.

Mehta, Mira. *Health through Yoga: Simple Practice Routines and a Guide to the Ancient Teachings*. London: Thorsons, 2002.

Monro, Dr. Robin, Dr. Nagarathna, and Dr. Nagendra. *Yoga for Common Ailments*. New York: Fireside, 1991.

Schiffman, Erich. *Yoga: The Spirit and Practice of Moving into Stillness*. New York: Pocket Books, 1996.

Sparrowe, Linda with Patricia Walden. *The Woman's Book of Yoga and Health: A Lifelong Guide to Wellness*. Boston: Shambhala Publications, 2002.

Yoga Sutras of Patanjali, as interpreted by Mukunda Stiles. Red Wheeler/Weiser Books, 2002.

Periodicals

Yoga International Magazine (bimonthly), Himalayan International Institute, RR1, Box 407, Honesdale, PA 18431; 800-822-4547; yimag.org

Yoga Journal (bimonthly), 2054 University Avenue, Berkeley, CA 94704; 800-600-9642; yogajournal.com

Yoga World (newsletter), Yoga Research and Education Center, 2400A County Center Drive, Santa Rosa, CA 95403; 707-566-9000; yogaworld.html

Web Sites

bksiyengar.com: Iyengar yoga official website

classicyoga.org/directory: Comprehensive directory of yoga resources

deeshan.com: Daily inspirational quotes about meditation

realization.org: Articles, interviews, resources, and links to many other related sites about yoga, meditation, and more

yoga.com: Comprehensive and easy to navigate. Has an online store that offers yoga clothing, videos, music, books, props, gifts; lists events, articles, and forums (women's health, meditation, beginners); also links to other sites

yogadirectory.com: Set up like a search engine so users can search by subject, which includes centers and organizations, books and periodicals, entertainment and media, healing and health, marketplace and products, references and resources, retreats, teachers and training, and yoga traditions

yogaforbeginners.com: Accessible website designed for those new to yoga; basic information about yoga; styles; resources

yogasite.com: "An eclectic collection of yoga connections," this site offers information about yoga poses and styles of yoga, yoga therapy information, breathing and meditation, Q&A, retreats, organizations, products, and a list of recent features

yoyoga.com: Fun, attractive, and informative site

Yoga Centers/Organizations

American Sanskrit Institute, Six Main St., Chester, CT 06412; 860-526-1532; americansanskrit.com. The institute offers classes for learning Sanskrit through an immersion experience, an online store where you can purchase books and mandalas, and an archive of writings by ASI director Vyaas Houston.

American Yoga Association, P.O. Box 19986, Sarasota, FL 34276; 941-927-4977; americanyogaassociation.org. Free yoga lessons are offered, as well as an online store of books and videotapes, and advice on how to select an instructor and start practicing yoga.

Himalayan International Institute of Yoga Science and Philosophy, P. O. Box 1127, Honesdale, PA 18431; 800-822-4547; himalayaninstitute.org. This organization sponsors workshops and retreats, has over 60 titles in print on yoga, guided meditation, and other topics, and publishes *Yoga International* magazine every other month.

International Association of Yoga Therapists, PO Box 2418, Sebastopol, CA 95473; 707-928-9898; iayt.org. The professional division of the Yoga Research and Education Center (see next page) devoted to yoga therapy and professional networking. Members receive subscriptions to the annual *International Journal of Yoga Therapy* and the triannual *Yoga Studies* newsletter, as well as access to IAYA's professional referral service.

International Yoga Teachers Association and Yoga for Health Foundation, 23 Morgan Street, Thornleigh NSW 2120 Australia. The International Yoga Teachers Association provides yoga teacher training and professional development. The Yoga for Health Foundation offers correspondence courses that specifically consider the yogic concept of the whole person and how it relates to human health.

Iyengar Yoga Institute, 223A Randolph Avenue, London W9 1NL; +44 (0)20-7624-3030; iyi.org.uk. Offers specialty classes for children and pregnant women, sponsors workshops (in the UK only) for teachers and practitioners, and sells many books and videos through the online store.

Kripalu Center for Yoga and Health, P.O. Box 793, Lenox, MA 02140; 800-741-7353, 413-448-3384; kripalu.org. Offers intensive summer courses, and publishes instructional videos and a cookbook for those interested in diet and nutrition.

Omega Institute for Holistic Studies, 150 Lake Drive, Rhinebeck, NY 12571; 845-266-4444; eomega.org. Provides education that is designed to improve health and well-being, promote creativity, and integrate mind, body, and spirit. Featured faculty members include Deepak Chopra, Wayne Dyer, Ralph Nader, and Alice Walker, among others.

Phoenix Rising Yoga Therapy, P.O. Box 819, Housatonic, MA 02136; 800-288-9642; pryt.com. Focuses on the therapeutic application of yoga, based on a completely holistic model, and offers courses to train healers. Web site will help you find a practitioner and features weekly yoga tips.

Sivananda Yoga Vedanta Center, 234 West 24th Street, New York, NY 10011; 52 Community Centre, East of Kailash, New Delhi 110065 India; sivananda.org/ny. Hosts special events and workshops, offers intensive courses for beginning and intermediate practitioners alike, and features special classes for prenatal and postpartum yoga, as well as vegetarian cooking workshops.

White Lotus Foundation, 2500 San Marcos Pass, Santa Barbara, CA 93105; 805-964-1944; whitelotus.org. Maintains a mountain retreat center near Santa Barbara, overlooking the Pacific Ocean, which features a library/media center and underground Hopi-style "Kiva" temple. Programs include teacher training, yoga retreats, and a weekend pranayama workshop.

Yoga Research and Education Center, 2400A County Center Drive, Santa Rosa, CA 95403; 707-566-9000; yrec.org. A non-profit tax-exempt corporation that serves yoga researchers, educators, and practitioners. Its staff and affiliates include professionals of medicine, education, psychology, philosophy, indology, and religion, and is committed to conserving the traditional yoga teachings.

Index

Acknowledgments

I would like to acknowledge the continual guidance, support, and assistance of my editor Leigh Anna Mendenhall, who envisioned this book and kept me focused and on track, as well as Nicole Kaufman, whose elegant and flowing illustrations grace the pages of *Essential Yoga*. Thanks to Jeff Durham for his diligent efforts in sleuthing the Sanskrit translations. I also wish to acknowledge yoga teacher Paul Howard for the endless supply of energy and enthusiasm that he brought to this project. Special thanks to my cheerleaders—Daryl Juran, Kathe Gregory, Maggie McNally, Peaco Todd—for their unceasing and unwavering support, optimism, and wisdom. Thanks, gratitude, and love to my family and friends, always the shining lights along my path. Finally, for his patience and devotion, special thanks to my husband, Ken Kevorkian.

Blessings to you all.